FIRE-RAISING: ITS MOTIVATION AND MANAGEMENT

WITHDRAWN

Fire – and in particular its misuse – has always had a fascination for certain people. In recent years fire-raising has become an increasing problem, in Britain and elsewhere, and the cost in both human and economic terms has risen sharply. The phenomenon is also known, in various parts of the world, as arson (the legal term), incendiarism, fire-setting and pyromania. The author has chosen to use the term 'fire-raising' because it is general enough to encompass all these other terms. *Fire-Raising* sets the phenomenon in an historical and anthropological context and analyses the extent of the problem.

Professor Herschel Prins draws on many research papers, published in a range of professional and academic journals, and brings their findings together in an accessible form. Although fire-raising is a complex matter, and the motives of fire-raisers equally complex, the clear guidance presented in this book will do much to inform all those involved in the investigation and management of people who use fire for unlawful purposes. It will be essential reading for a wide range of individuals who deal with this problem – fire-service staff, police, medical professionals of various kinds, criminologists, as well as psychiatrists, social workers, lawyers, magistrates and judges.

Herschel Prins is a professor at the Midlands Centre for Criminology and Criminal Justice, University of Loughborough, and Visiting Professor in Clinical Criminology, Nottingham Trent University.

WITHDRAWN

BY THE SAME AUTHOR

OFFENDERS, DEVIANTS OR PATIENTS
An introduction to the study of socio-forensic problems
Tavistock, 1980

CRIMINAL BEHAVIOUR
An introduction to criminology and the penal system
Second edition
Tavistock, 1982

DANGEROUS BEHAVIOUR, THE LAW AND MENTAL
DISORDER
Tavistock, 1986

BIZARRE BEHAVIOURS
Tavistock/Routledge, 1990

FIRE-RAISING: ITS MOTIVATION AND MANAGEMENT

WITHDRAWN

Herschel Prins

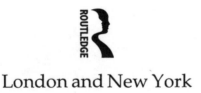

London and New York

First published in 1994
by Routledge
11 New Fetter Lane, London EC4P 4EE

Simultaneously published in the USA and Canada
by Routledge
29 West 35th Street, New York, NY 10001

© 1994 Herschel Prins

Typeset in Palatino
by LaserScript Limited, Mitcham, Surrey
Printed and bound in Great Britain by
Biddles Ltd, Guildford and King's Lynn

British Library Cataloguing in Publication Data
A catalogue record for this book is available from the British Library.

Library of Congress Cataloging in Publication Data
Prins, Herschel A.
Fire-raising: its motivation and management/Herschel Prins.
p. cm.
Includes bibliographical references and index.
1. Arson–Psychological aspects. 2. Arson–Prevention.
I. Title.
RC569.5.P9P75 1994   93-7385
616.85'845–dc20   CIP
ISBN 0–415–05984–4 (hbk)
ISBN 0–415–05985–2 (pbk)

'Fire is a good servant but a bad master.'
Seventeenth-century proverb

'There are few delinquencies as wayward as fire-raising that will have attracted those of us who count ourselves as law abiding. The almost universal fascination with fire, the awareness of both its comfort and its destructiveness, set the context in which this admirably clear book looks at those for whom this everyday enchantment has turned to pathological expression. Drawing widely on anthropology, psychology and the author's renowned expertise in clinical criminology, Herschel Prins offers a notably accessible consideration of the facts and theories that accompany the study of fire-raising. Case studies and vignettes serve to capture further the various dynamics and motivations that underlie what is one of the least easily understood of the deviant behaviours.

What comes across so clearly from this book is the sheer complexity of fire-raising as something that is adopted by a whole range of distressed, dissatisfied or just plain disagreeable people. By acknowledging this variety, Herschel Prins has given us a comprehensive, thoroughly readable and refreshingly informative summary of how best to understand and manage the fire-raiser.'

Professor David Webb,
Head of the Department of Applied Social Studies,
Nottingham Trent University

'Herschel Prins can always be relied on to give a lucid and measured account of his subject. He assembles his material with meticulous care and professional rigour. This book will enlighten the general reader but also provide a sound introduction to those professionally involved in any aspect of this serious and growing problem. A wide range of services and public bodies are affected by what can be a terrifying and extremely costly destructive act. We need to understand much more about its motivation and develop strategies of prevention and containment. This is not a problem which can just be left for the "fire-fighters" to deal with.

Herschel Prins shares his own fascination for what has always been a peculiarly potent symbol for mankind and helps the reader to comprehend how this natural force provides accessible and destructive power on a bewildering scale. An incident of school burning with one disaffected pupil acting out resentment at the cost of millions of pounds makes the point. It is in all our interests to have a better understanding of behaviour which can have such ravaging consequences. Herschel Prins has made an important contribution to that.'

Sir Michael Day OBE

CONTENTS

ILLUSTRATIONS

FIGURES

TABLES

ACKNOWLEDGEMENTS

A number of individuals and organisations have assisted me in the preparation of this book. I am grateful to Mr R.D. Mackay, Reader in Criminal Law, Department of Law, De Montfort University, Leicester, for assistance with the legal matters referred to in Chapter 3; to Mr Rodger Ide of the Home Office Forensic Science Service for kindly looking at and commenting upon Chapter 4. The Fire Protection Association and Mr J.C. Munro of the Association of British Insurers supplied helpful data as did Mr M. Butwell of the Special Hospitals Service Authority. I am grateful to the Fire and Emergency Planning Department of the Home Office for permission to use the tables and figures reproduced in Chapters 3 and 5. My continuing thanks to Mrs Janet Kirkwood for preparing such good 'copy' from my mutilated drafts and to my wife, Norma, for once again spotting grammatical and other errors – and putting them right! Finally, my warm thanks are due to Edwina Welham, my editor at Routledge, for tolerating a series of delays in the preparation and final submission of the manuscript with a great deal of patience and good humour. If this book has any merit, it is due to all the kindly disposed individuals and organisations mentioned above. However, they are in no way responsible for my errors, omissions and misinterpretations.

Houghton on the Hill,
Leicestershire,
May 1993

1

PREAMBLE

'How great a little fire doth kindleth'
James 3: 5

As I shall show in Chapter 2, the phenomenon of fire has always played a significant and many-faceted part in the history of humanity. Throughout this history it has been put to many uses; for example as an agent of succour, warmth and light, of healing and cleansing, but also of destruction. This last capacity is only all too self-evident in contemporary society with almost daily reports of bombings, explosions and serious accidents involving deaths and maimings caused by fire. However, the fortunes amassed from the manufacture of explosive substances some-times may be put to good use, as for example in the case of Alfred Nobel. There are few rituals in which it has not played a sig-nificant part. In this context, Mary Douglas, the distinguished anthropologist, makes the following important point:

> Death, blood and coldness are confronted by their oppo-sites, life, sex and fire. All six powers are dangerous. The three positive powers are dangerous unless separated from one another and are in danger from contact with death, blood or coldness.[1]

In addition, fire, as a phenomenon, has held, and continues to hold, a fascination every bit as powerful as that evoked by life and death. This universal fascination and its legacy have import-ant implications for those who work in various capacities with individuals who use fire for destructive and unlawful purposes. In this small book I shall be concerned, mainly, with some of these more worrying aspects and with the complex motives of

1

those who seek to use it in this way. In order to do this it will be necessary to examine the phenomenon briefly in its cultural and historical context; this is done in Chapter 2. Thereafter we can then proceed in the remaining chapters to examine the current prevalence of fire-raising, some legal aspects, outline some of the methods used in its investigation, offer some analyses of the kind of people who raise fires, speculate about their motives and suggest how their behaviour might be best managed and controlled.

A word of explanation is necessary concerning the choice of title for this book – *Fire-Raising*. The phenomenon is also known (in various parts of the world) as arson (the *legal* term used), incendiarism, fire-setting (terms favoured in the USA and Canada), pyromania (a restricted description once favoured in the nineteenth century and used to denote a form of insanity) and pathological fire-setting (a term used to indicate the involvement of abnormal mental states). I have chosen to use the term 'fire-raising' as being general enough to encompass all these other terms and to embrace the various aspects of the phenomena to be discussed. It is hoped that this device will be acceptable to a wide (and, hopefully, international) readership.

As I shall demonstrate, fire-raising is a very worrying form of behaviour. Not only is its detection difficult, but the harm caused to both persons and property can be considerable. As we shall see in Chapter 3, statistics indicate that fires of 'doubtful origin' or 'malicious ignition' (to use the terms preferred by the fire-service authorities) and arson (the legal description) have been increasing considerably in both the UK and the USA in recent years.

A wide range of professionals are likely to be involved in making judgements about the past and possible future behaviour of those involved in, or convicted of, setting fires (for example, courts at all levels; parole and other discharge authorities; probation and social service personnel – field and residential; the police; and penal and health care staff of various kinds). For this reason it is hoped that this book will appeal to both students and experienced workers in all these disciplines. In addition, I hope also it will be of value to the 'interested reader' who may wish to improve his or her knowledge of the topic; for, sadly, the 'interested reader' may all too often be the subject of a fire-raiser's attentions. There are numerous articles in a variety of professional journals on the subject, but some are not readily available to students, busy professionals or the general reader.

A further word here is in order on the focus and structure of the book. The structure and content of Chapters 1 to 4 should be self-evident. In effect, they set the scene for the material in Chapters 5 to 7. Chapters 5 and 6 deal with both motivation and management in adults and children respectively. One approach would have been to have dealt with the motivations of these two groups together and then have dealt with management separately. In my view this would have been an artificial and unhelpful distinction since management must, perforce, be dependent upon motivation and attitudes. The wider aspects of motivation are dealt with in Chapter 7. Put another way, the material in Chapters 5 and 6 deals with the problem at the micro-level and that in Chapter 7 at the macro-level. Both are equally important if the problem of fire-raising is to be addressed adequately and dealt with.

This book is not intended as a manual by which professionals will find sure and certain answers to the problems of management of individual cases. In the present state of our knowledge and skills any attempt to do so would be foolhardy and professionally arrogant. Its purpose rather is to offer a framework and a synthesis of thinking and practice with which a variety of professionals and others can not only chart their own course of study and action but, it is to be hoped, develop their thinking from where I have left off. There are very few books of recent date that deal to any great extent with the motivation of fire-raisers; notable exceptions being the works by Scott and Canter in this country and by Macdonald and Wooden and Berkey in the USA.[2] I hope, therefore, that this modest work will help to fill a gap in the existing literature.

2

CONTEXT

'The wise man does not discriminate; he gathers together all the
shreds of light from wherever they may come.'

Umberto Eco, *Foucault's Pendulum*

BRIEF HISTORICAL COMMENT

The universal phenomenon of fire is well documented.
Bronowski, in his scientific and literary *tour de force, The Ascent of
Man*, states that 'Fire has been known to early man for about four
hundred thousand years, we think. That implies that fire had
already been discovered by Homo erectus.'[1] Fire is a powerful
symbol, as is evident from a consideration of mythology. For
example, in ancient Egyptian myth, the Phoenix was said to live
for hundreds of years, burn itself to death and then rise again
from the ashes of its funeral pyre – an association between fire
and life eternal that is echoed in the perpetual flames that burn at
national war memorials to those fallen in battle. This legend of
birth, death and rebirth appears to have a universal fascination
for it demonstrates parallels with the myths surrounding the
re-creation of life as exemplified in the form of Frankenstein's
Monster. It also appears in the ubiquitous life and death myth of
the vampire, the subject of numerous novels, films and plays.[2] In
Greek mythology, as we shall see, Prometheus, having stolen fire
from the Gods, was condemned to the everlasting torment of
having his liver torn out by vultures. In less mythical and more
practical fashion it is interesting to note here that the Greeks also
used fire for the destruction of the bodies of those who had taken
their own lives. (They also cut off the hand by which the suicides

4

had killed themselves and buried it separately.) Roman culture also had a 'goddess of the domestic hearth named Vesta, who, in due course, was worshipped in a temple tended by virgin priestesses'.[3]

There are numerous references to fire, its uses and abuses, in the Bible and it also appears in liturgical practice. God revealed himself to Moses in the burning bush and the Book of Exodus recounts how fire guided the Israelites by night through the wilderness: 'all the time the Lord went before them, by day a pillar of cloud . . . by night a pillar of fire to give them light, so that they could travel by night and day' (13: 21–2). Fire was also used as an indication of the presence of the Divine and as a symbol of direction to Moses when the Angel of the Lord appeared to him in the burning bush (Exodus 3: 2). Fire was of course also used for sacrificial purposes – sometimes to the point of human sacrifice, as in the case of Abraham and his son Isaac, for he 'bound . . . Isaac and laid him on the altar on top of the wood' (Genesis, 22: 9) – a sore test of faith. Fire was also associated with notions of punishment. In the book of Deuteronomy we find the words 'The Lord thy God is a consuming fire, even a jealous God' (4: 24). We also find reference to fire's use for purposes of revenge. Topp cites the illustration of the children of Judah putting Jerusalem to the sword and then firing it (Judges, 1: 8).[4] Samson took revenge on his father-in-law by destroying his harvest by fire (Judges, 15: 6). The use of fire for purposes of revenge is an important topic and one I shall return to in discussing clinical examples of fire-raising.

In the Christian era fire is represented in somewhat different terms, markedly as a form of punishment for the souls of the damned and as a purifying force to be harnessed on behalf of those seeking the righteous life. However, it was its former purpose that no doubt provided the catalyst for the use of fire for the burning of heretics and witches.[5] Perhaps one of the most notable people to have suffered in this way was the semi-legendary St Joan of Arc, as a result of her activities in leading the French against the English. In the years that were to follow, history was to record innumerable instances of clerics and others being burned at the stake. It would be erroneous to think that such barbaric activity was limited to Christian/Western culture, however. In the Hindu religion, its use in admittedly less overt punishing form can be seen in the practice of *Suttee* – the highly symbolic self-immolation performed by widows on the funeral pyres of their husbands. Self-immolation is also seen in myth and legend, as for example in the manner in which Brünhilde dies on the massive funeral pyre in the final scene of Wagner's opera *Götterdämmerung*.

Both Freud and Jung made use of the legend of Prometheus in connection with their attempts to understand fire as a phenomenon. In brief, they considered that Prometheus needed to outwit the Gods by stealing fire from them. It is said that, in so doing, he transported it in a hollow stick. This, they suggested, could be viewed at one and the same time as both a male and female symbol of sexuality. Implicit in this was said to be a degree of role and identity confusion – a characteristic, as we shall see later, sometimes found in those who indulge in fire-raising. It has already been noted that Prometheus was punished for his crime in a particularly unpleasant fashion, demonstrating since earliest times the implied risks in handling potentially dangerous forces such as fire and sex. There are other Greek mythical references to fire. There is the famous legend of how Phaethon, son of the Sun God Helios and of the nymph Clymene, insisted on driving his father's chariot for a day. Being unskilled, he drove the chariot so close to the earth that he burned it. The God Zeus, concerned that this inexperienced youth might do further damage, directed a thunderbolt at the chariot, killing Phaethon. There is also the legend of Icarus, the son of Daedalus. Icarus attempted to flee from imprisonment by King Minos on wings fashioned by his father. However, the sun melted them and he perished. These myths merely add to the injunctions about the risks of unleashing potentionally dangerous forces such as fire.

FIRE AND MAGICAL BELIEFS

Some of the most interesting, if somewhat dated, accounts of the magical beliefs associated with fire common amongst so-called primitive peoples are to be found in the writings of the great pioneer anthropologist Sir James George Frazer.[6] His findings, gathered over many years, led him to suggest, for example, that it was considered that health, luck and indeed life could be secured by gathering the cactus plant, supposedly the gourd of the Gods of Fire. He discovered a number of ceremonies that were used to relieve women, in particular, of sin through the use of fire. In

Timor, he found that in times of war the High Priest never left the temple so that the fire could be kept burning. If he were to leave, it was believed that disaster might befall the warriors. In other parts of the world he discovered the belief that the priests were endowed with the power to raise both fire and storm. He reports a number of other instances of the magical belief in the power of fire. For example, he describes the belief that flood rains could be stopped by burning the branch of a certain tree in the desert and then sprinkling the branch with water. This was said to reduce the rainfall. In other parts, in order to *produce* rain, the village head-man was said to place a burning banch on the grave of a man who had died of burns. He would then guard the branch while he prayed that rain would fall. Frazer considered that in this type of situation the extinguishing of the fire with water, which is an imitation of rain, was reinforced by the influence of the dead man, who, having been burned to death, would naturally be anxious for the descent of rain to cool his sacred body and assuage his pains.[7] One supposes that the purpose was, no doubt, to propitiate the Gods in order to evoke beneficial outcomes by means of the phenomenon of 'sympathetic magic'.

Frazer devotes a good deal of space to the provision of highly detailed accounts of various forms of fire festivals (rituals) that have existed since very early times throughout Europe and elsewhere. A number of European rituals take place at Hallowe'en, on Christmas Day and on the twelfth day after Christmas. Various suggestions are offered as to the purposes of their existence. They include the securing of good crops, good health, a happy marriage increased the prevention of fertility and the effect of witchcraft. Some of these rituals also appear to have their less pleasant elements; for example, the burning alive of cats while shepherds danced their flocks through the smoke and flames as a means of guarding against sickness and witchcraft. In these rituals there also seems to have been an element of 'playing with fire'. This is illustrated by the practice adopted by some young people of dancing over the embers to see who could avoid being burned by them. It is said that those who were successful would be married within the year! Another interesting custom is of possible significance in relation to the later practice of burning witches. This involved the burning of straw men on which it is said the local inhabitants projected all their sins and thus purged themselves. Frazer makes particular comment upon the phenomenon of Easter Fires – said to be of pagan character and origin. He states:

> The fires are always kindled, year after year, on the same hill, which accordingly often takes the name of Easter Mountain. It is a fine spectacle to watch from some eminence, the bonfires flaring up one after another in the neighbouring heights . . . in the belief of the peasants, the fields will be fruitful . . . and their houses will be safe from conflagration or sickness.[8]

Frazer made an important distinction between what he described as 'need-fires' and other types of fire. The former tended to exist for life-preserving and purificatory purposes, though one finds in his accounts that the distinction is not always as clear-cut as this.

Similar fire phenomena have been described more recently by the British folklore authority Christina Hole.[9] For example, she describes the practice of 'Burning the Old Year Out' in various places in Scotland; from her descriptions this practice seems to serve purposes very similar to those rituals described by Frazer. She also describes a very interesting event that takes place on New Year's Eve at Allendale in Northumberland. A procession is formed, in which those taking part carry blazing half-barrels of tar and other combustible materials on their heads. This head-gear is then thrown, in processional fashion, onto a central bonfire. Immediately after midnight, the procession sets off to 'first-foot' round the parish. Hole reports that in days gone by 'open house was kept for all and sundry', but 'so many strangers now come to witness the ceremony that it is no longer possible'.[10] A similar practice was 'Burning the Clavie', which took place in Morayshire, Scotland, and is said to have ensured good luck for the year.[11] (p.50). It is interesting to note that in this particular ceremony no stranger could take part and the tools used were given or borrowed, not bought. The use of a metal hammer in the preparations was expressly forbidden. One supposes that these precautions were intended to preserve purity. A similar practice existed in Herefordshire and in Worcestershire – known in those parts as 'Burning the Bush'.

It has only been possible to touch upon a minute aspect of the fascinating phenomena described by Frazer and Hole. Both these writers (but Frazer in particular) described these phenomena in considerable detail; the reader interested in pursuing this anthropological and folklore background should consult these works for this and much other fascinating information.

MORE RECENT HISTORY

The deliberately destructive use of fire in its various forms is of course well documented in history. There are very early references to the use of mixtures of the chemicals potassium nitrate, charcoal and sulphur for making crude bombing devices. Macdonald notes that Leonardo da Vinci made sketches for the preparation of mortars.[12] In the sixteenth century there are descriptions of various complicated 'noxious engines' that used explosive devices to cause horrifying injuries to those within range. Readers of this book will need no reminder of the details of the Gunpowder Plot of November 5, 1605. In more recent years, it is sad to record that, in so-called civilised communities, more and more ingenious methods have been discovered by the technicians of terrorism to cause carnage and mayhem. It should be noted here that the main thrust of this small work is about fire-raising specifically, and I have made a somewhat artificial, but I think justifiable, distinction between this and bombing and terrorist activities. The latter topics receive some passing reference in later chapters but require more specific and detailed treatment than I can afford. Useful accounts may be found in Macdonald's book *Bombers and Firesetters*.[13]

MEDICAL INTEREST IN THE TOPIC

Fire has, of course, a long history of medical usage, notably for purposes of cauterisation. Scott suggests that the Greek physician Hippocrates was well aware of the advantages of cauterisation when he stated that 'what medicine does not cure then the iron does . . . and what the iron does not cure fire exterminates.'[14] He also quotes the early physician Paré who pointed out the disadvantages of such draconian treatment: 'Nature must regenerate a new flesh instead of that which hath been burnt, as also the bones remaines discovered and bare; and by this means from the most part there remains an ulcer incurable.'[15]

In the middle of the nineteenth century (and possibly earlier) physicians began to turn their attention and interest towards what were regarded as pathological forms of fire-raising. (See further discussion in Chapters 5 and 6.) The term 'pyromania' was probably first introduced at about this time by the French physician Marc. Soon afterwards, German physicians were to develop this interest further. They suggested that these particular forms of fire-raising were most frequently found in sexually frustrated and rather dull teenage country girls. Such statements would rightly be criticised today by those interested in, and informed about, gender issues. The German physicians also suggested that the condition was occasionally seen in older men where it appeared to be associated with orgiastic satisfaction. This association between fire and sexuality was, as we have already noted, later developed within the context of the myth of Prometheus, notably by Freud and later by Jung, who viewed it as a symbolic and archetypical outlet for sexual impulses. Currently, somewhat less extreme psychoanalytic interpretations of its complex basis prevail, but, as we shall see when we examine the motivations of fire-raisers more closely, there are certainly some cases in which a specific association between fire and sexuality appears to be of importance.

With this brief context-setting review in mind we can now turn our attention to the current size of the problem and some legal aspects.

3

THE SIZE OF THE PROBLEM AND LEGAL ASPECTS

'There are three kinds of lies; lies, damned lies, and statistics.'

Mark Twain

INTRODUCTION

In recent years concern about the increase in the number of fires from various causes has been expressed by authorities thoughout the world. In this chapter, I shall attempt to demonstrate this increase from various sources and to make the point that fires caused by arson (see later for legal definition) and fires from other causes (such as deliberate or non-accidental ignition) need to be viewed together in order to obtain an accurate total picture.

In the UK, the Home Office has been concerned for a number of years about fires caused by vandalism and a working party was established to examine this problem. This working party (chaired by Mr G.T. Rudd) reported in 1980.[1] The members of the working party stressed the difficulty of measuring the size of the problem accurately and, in particular, making comparisons between offences recorded as arson and those identified by the various fire service authorities as fires of 'malicious' ignition or doubtful origin!

This problem remains; because of it, a good deal of caution should be exercised in interpreting the figures quoted later in this chapter. This is even more important when trying to make cross-country comparisons. Mark Twain's cautionary comment cited at the beginning of this chapter needs to be uppermost in the reader's mind when reviewing the figures quoted below. As already indicated, it is notoriously difficult to obtain adequate and accurate base-line data and this is a particularly acute

11

problem at international level and even between cities and states in the *same* country (as, for example, in the USA). The figures quoted here may give the appearance of having been chosen for citation in a somewhat arbitrary fashion. However, this is not the case. They have been chosen on the basis of being the best data available and being representative of trends over a reasonable time span. Finally, the true picture at any particular moment is always elusive because figures inevitably become outdated during the period of their compilation and publication.

However, it does appear that even if we allow for all these difficulties of collation, recording and interpretation, the number of cases of arson and fires caused by 'malicious ignition' or of 'doubtful origin' is greater than the *published* figures would suggest. Numerous and varied sources have been used for the figures quoted later, which are identified and acknowledged in the notes and references at the end of the book. It is possible that the increase in non-accidental fires can be seen as part of the problem of the increase in violence against persons and property in general. In a recent interesting paper, Palermo *et al.*[2] note the worrying increase in violence in the USA. They indicate that 2 million serious victimisations were reported in 1984 and that the estimated current cost to victims is in the region of many billions of dollars annually. They make particular comment on the increase in reported crimes of violence in the Metropolitan area of London in 1987. These show an 11 per cent increase over those reported in 1986 and a 26 per cent increase in 1988. They indicate that perpetrators of such crimes are predominantly young adult males. It is relevant to note that, as I shall show later, arson is a crime committed predominantly by young adult males: 93 per cent of those convicted of arson are male and 61 per cent are under 21.[3] It would be unwise to make too much of the possible links between arson (as violence against property) and other types of violence, but it may reflect a continuing and disturbing trend. Such a trend is illustrated in some recent observations by the well respected psychiatrist Anthony Storr:

> I think that *Homo Sapiens* has not altered very much in fundamental physical or psychological characteristics since he first appeared upon the scene; and that the best we can hope for is some slight modification of his nastier traits of personality in the light of increased understanding.[4]

GENERAL STATISTICAL OBSERVATIONS

In a wide-ranging review of the topic, Woodward[5] noted that the numbers of malicious fires in buildings had increased fourfold from 1956 to 1964 and that the position was getting steadily worse. He observed that

> world-wide it can be said that the cost of arson as a proportion of all costs of fire is at least fifteen per cent and can be as high as fifty per cent depending on the country . . . fire insurers thoughout the world are having to devote between one quarter and a third of their total loss expenditure to pay for fire losses resulting from arson.[6]

He also quotes evidence from the Gerling Institute of Cologne that there had been an '"alarming increase" in the number of deliberately started fires as reflected in the criminal statistics of all industrial countries'.[7] (see Table 3.1)

It is important to note that although the *total* number of fires for the period cited in Table 3.1 did not fluctuate markedly, the *percentage* adjudged to be of malicious ignition rose more than sixfold.

Woodward also reports similar percentage increases in 'large fires'[8] in the UK for the same periods (see Table 3.2).

Criminal statistics: England and Wales

From the criminal statistics for England and Wales one can see a steady increase in the number of recorded cases of arson and criminal damage endangering life (Table 3.3: see later for legal definitions).[9]

Table 3.1 Incidents of malicious fire-raising in buildings (excluding dwellings) as a percentage of total fires in the UK, 1964–84

Year	Malicious ignition	Total fires	Percentage
1964	1,900	40,000	4.8
1974	6,160	46,381	13.3
1984	11,396	42,574	26.8

Source: C.D. Woodward, 'Arson: The Major Fire Problem of the 1980s', *Journal of the Society of Fellows. The Chartered Insurance Institute*, Vol. 2 (Pt 1), 1987, p. 56.

Table 3.2 Incidents of malicious fire-raising as a percentage of total
'large fires ' in the UK, 1964–84

Year	Malicious ignition	Total fires	Percentage
1964	37	658	5.6
1974	334	1,210	27.6
1984	393	1,029	38.2

Source: Woodward, op. cit., p. 56.

A more detailed analysis of the manner in which the courts
dealt with cases of arson in the year 1986 may be seen from Tables
3.4 and 3.5. In that year 47 per cent of arson cases were dealt with
by magistrates courts and 53 per cent by crown courts.

Each year a small number of persons convicted of arson are
dealt with by way of mental health disposals; such disposals are
given further consideration in later chapters. In 1987, 29 persons
(16 males and 13 females) were admitted to one or other of the
three special (high security) hospitals in England and Wales
(Broadmoor, Rampton and Ashworth).[10] However, when one
examines the figures for *all patients* currently detained in these
hospitals (some 1,700) who are past offenders, the figure is much
higher – about 550. Still, this figure includes not only persons sent
to the hospitals under court order for an index offence or arson,
but also those who may be detained there under the civil powers
of the Mental Health Act, 1983 (or its predecessor, the Act of
1959), or for assessment purposes, or on transfer from prison
either during remand or following sentence. The figures for
admissions for the years 1983 to 1987 are given in Table 3.6.

Table 3.3 Persons found guilty of or cautioned for arson and criminal
damage endangering life, England and Wales, 1982–90

	1982	1984	1986	1988	1990
Arson	3,270	3,730	2,881	3,167	3,393
Criminal damage endangering life	45	64	74	93	85

Sources: H. Prins, *Dangerous Behaviour, the Law and Mental Disorder*, London,
Tavistock, 1986, p. 213; Woodward, op. cit., p. 56; Home Office, *Criminal Statistics
for England and Wales*, 1990, Cm 1935, London, HMSO, 1992, Table 5.18, p. 124.

Table 3.4 Proportionate use of different types of sentence for arson by type of court in England and Wales, 1986

Sentence	Magistrates court (%)	Crown court (%)
Discharge	22	–
Probation order	11	15
Attendance centre order	10	–
Supervision order	15	–
Community service order	6	6
Fine	15	1
Care order	3	–
Suspended sentence	2	9
Immediate custody	11	61
Mental Health Act 1983	–	5
Other	5	3

Source: Home Office, *Standing Conference on Crime Prevention: Report of the Working Group on the Prevention of Arson*, December 6, 1988, p. 40.

Table 3.5 Lengths of immediate custodial sentences imposed by the crown court in England and Wales, 1986, for arson and for all offences

Sentence length	Proportion for arson (%)	Proportion for all offences (%)
Up to 4 months	1	17
Over 4 months to 6 months	3	15
Over 6 months to 12 months	11	26
Over 12 months to 18 months	15	14
Over 18 months to 2 years	18	9
Over 2 years to 3 years	27	9
Over 3 years to 4 years	11	4
Over 4 years to 5 years	7	2
Over 5 years to 7 years	2	2
Over 7 years	5	2

Source: Home Office, *Report of the Working Group on the Prevention of Arson*, op. cit., p. 40. (Reproduced with permission.)

15

Table 3.6 Admissions for arson to special hospitals in England and Wales, 1983–7

	1983	1984	1985	1986	1987
Male	11	15	21	17	16
Female	6	11	19	14	13
Total	17	26	40	31	29

Source: Mr M. Butwell, Special Hospitals Service Authority, personal communication, January 12, 1991.

It is interesting to note the high proportion of females to males admitted. Serious cases of arson involving a mental disorder sufficient to satisfy the stringent criteria of the Mental Health Act, 1983, seem fairly equally divided between the sexes – unlike some other offences. Of the total number of patients detained and referred to in Table 3.6, 33 per cent were diagnosed as suffering from *mental illness*, 43 per cent from *personality disorder*, and the remainder from *mental impairment, severe mental impairment* or a combination of *mental impairment with mental illness or personality disorder.* The patients were distributed fairly equally between the three hospitals with a slightly increased proportion at Rampton.[11] It should be noted that the figures quoted in Table 3.6 refer only to those offender-patients whose behaviour was judged to be sufficiently dangerous to justify admission to a *high security* hospital. A small number of psychiatrically disturbed arsonists may be dealt with by other means of psychiatric disposal such as a probation order with a requirement for mental treatment under the Powers of Criminal Courts Act, 1973, as amended by the Criminal Justice Act, 1991.

A more detailed breakdown of the number of notifiable offences of arson reported by the police and the courts, and the numbers proceeded against, is shown in Figure 3.1. Figures 3.2 and 3.3 show the numbers of deliberate/possibly deliberate fires in the UK for the period 1978 to 1986. Some of this increase is no doubt attributable to improvements in the forensic detection of possible arson, but a substantial part is no doubt due to an actual increase in the incidence of the crime.

Figure 3.4 and Table 3.7 show the locations of all deliberate or possibly deliberate fires in occupied buildings in the UK in 1986 and for the years 1982 to 1986 respectively.

16

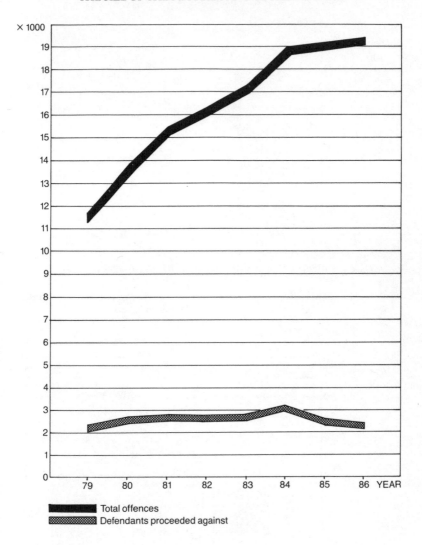

Figure 3.1 Notifiable offences of arson in England and Wales, 1979–86
Source: Home Office, *Report of the Working Group on the Prevention of Arson*, op. cit., p. 20. (Reproduced with permission.)

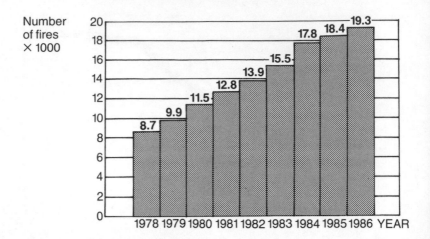

Figure 3.2 Deliberate or possibly deliberate fires in occupied buildings in the UK, 1979–86

Source: Home Office, *Report of the Working Group on the Prevention of Arson*, op. cit., p. 18. (Reproduced with permission.)

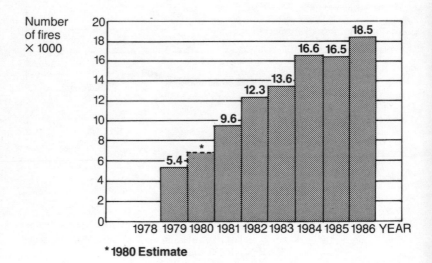

Figure 3.3 Deliberate or possibly deliberate fires in vehicles and other locations outdoors in the UK, 1979–86

Source: Home Office, *Report of the Working Group on the Prevention of Arson*, op. cit., p. 18. (Reproduced with permission.)

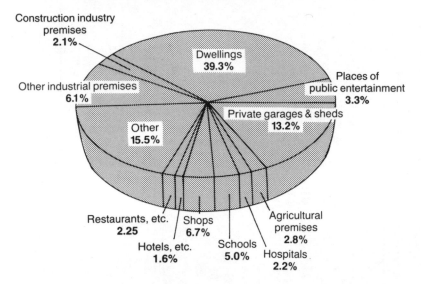

Figure 3.4 Locations of all deliberate or possibly deliberate fires in occupied buildings in the UK, 1986

Source: Home Office, *Report of the Working Group on the Prevention of Arson*, op. cit., p. 28. (Reproduced with permission.)

The financial cost of deliberate fire-raising

It has been calculated that in schools, 80 per cent of the fires which cause more that £50,000 of damage are deliberate. Every week, 40 schools are said to be seriously damaged by fire and one of these blazes may cost as much as £250,000. In 1986, as reported in *The Independent* (August 13, 1987, p. 11), the cost of arson in schools was said to be in excess of £150 million. In the same article, reference is made not just to the financial and economic costs, but to the traumatic impact on the children (particularly primary school children). One teacher is quoted as saying 'Some of the little ones were crying when they saw the remains of the building.' I shall be considering motivation in young people in considerable detail subsequently, but it is relevant to mention here one or two aspects in order to bring alive the mainly statistical presentation in this chapter.

In the article referred to above there is a description of how two teenage girls set fire to a school in Cheshire. They gave as their reason that they were harbouring a grudge because their teachers

Table 3.7 Locations of all deliberate or possibly deliberate fires in occupied buildings in the UK, 1982–6

Occupied buildings	1982	1983	1984	1985	1986
Dwellings	5,010	5,654	6,460	7,174	7,595
Private garages, sheds	1,739	1,906	2,244	2,176	2,545
Agricultural premises	431	423	505	501	541
Construction industry premises	358	349	401	364	401
Other industrial premises	1,001	1,014	1,310	1,245	1,181
Hospitals	403	449	399	410	433
Schools	864	926	1,108	1,012	972
Shops	932	1,124	1,256	1,254	1,299
Hotels, hostels, boarding houses	238	251	252	296	304
Restaurants, clubs, pubs	322	352	409	393	422
Places of public entertainment	527	596	695	666	637
Other or unspecified in occupied buildings	2,116	2,442	2,717	2,923	2,987
Other locations					
Road vehicles	9,780	10,623	12,481	12,756	14,578
Outdoor machinery and equipment	700	810	1,092	1,005	1,013
Other outdoor (excluding secondary fires)	1,844	2,171	3,046	2,694	2,871

Source: Home Office, *Report of the Working Group on the Prevention of Arson,* op. cit., p. 28. (Reproduced with permission.)

had failed to recognise sooner that they had been the victims of sexual abuse when younger. However, fire-raising in school is more often the work of teenage boys, mainly in the inner cities; their fire-raising is linked to other anti-social conduct. Vanity and vengeance may also play a part. A warped satisfaction might be derived from ransacking and then firing the building which may have provided the one real and possibly unhappy experience of authority in their lives. One of the main reasons that there are so few fatalities in deliberate fires in schools is that they usually occur at night. However, there have been some tragic incidents where young fire-raisers have been seriously injured as a result of their activities. In a later chapter I shall consider some measures that are being taken to prevent fire-raising in schools – and in other places.

To return to the cost of fires more generally, the Association of British Fire Insurers has indicated that a £1 million fire claim is not an uncommon occurrence today. Twenty-six fires costing more than £1 million took place in the period April–June 1990; and fire damage claims jumped to £239.3 million in the same quarter in 1989, an increase of 19 per cent. The Association lists 26 fires in the UK where the costs to insurers were in excess of £1 million; one being £16 million, one for £8 million and ten for £3 million and above.[12]

A recent development

Recently, there appears to have been a marked increase in a particular form of damage by fire; namely fires in various types of vehicles. Confirmation of this surmise is to be found in the returns in the *Fire Statistics for 1988*:

> In 1988, the year on year increases in road vehicle fires were halted by a slight fall of just over one per cent compared with 1987 to 49,000. The decrease was confined to accidental fires which fell by nearly 3 per cent for 1987 to 33,800.[13]

Road vehicle fires that were deliberate, or possibly deliberate, continued to show an increase; they accounted for 31 per cent of all fires in road vehicles in 1988 (15,212) compared with 9 per cent (2,439) in 1978. However, concerning *car* fires specifically, there was a small decrease (about 2 per cent) in 1988 compared with the figures for 1987.

It is not easy to suggest clear reasons for this disturbing trend of deliberate/possibly deliberate road vehicle fires. It may be merely a part of the general picture of vandalism referred to earlier – a desire to take out one's dissatisfaction on others better favoured by fortune. It may be a more frequently used method of avoiding detection for taking a vehicle without the owner's consent (TWOC); fire will of course destroy fingerprints. However, this seems a somewhat drastic method of escaping detection and is also one fraught with danger for the thief or thieves. An additional explanation has been afforded by the insurance world. Mr Robert Mead, Chairman of the Essex Branch of the British Insurance and Investment Brokers' Association, considers that the current recession may be partly responsible: 'If you have been made redundant and can't afford to keep your car, but can't sell it either, the temptation is there to report it stolen and set fire to it, or to get someone to do it for you.' Mr Mead anticipated, as a result of such fires and increased thefts from cars, that insurance premiums would rise – as indeed they have (*The Independent*, May 12, 1992, p. 4).

Deaths and other casualties from fires[14]

Deaths from fires in the UK fell very slightly from 929 in 1987 to 915 in 1988 – the lowest total since 1984. But within this total the number of deaths from fires in *dwellings* increased from 710 in 1987 to 732 in 1988. Such statistics will vary, of course, from year to year depending upon the number of 'disasters' that occur (for example, such events as Lockerbie, Kegworth and the fire at King's Cross, London). Non-fatal casualties[15] increased by just over 6 per cent from 12,600 in 1987 to nearly 13,400 in 1988 – a new peak.

THE INTERNATIONAL PICTURE

As already indicated, there appears to be an increase world-wide in fires, both accidental and deliberate. Some selected statistics are given below which serve to support this contention. However, the caution given earlier about making comparisons between countries must be repeated; there are considerable variations in the manner in which causes of fires are identified and in the collection and presentation of data.

United States

It has been reported that 'arson and suspected arson constitute the largest single cause of property damage due to fire in the United States' (National Fire Protection Association).[16] In 1988, such fires accounted for over $1.5 billion lost to fire in structural damage and $150 million lost to fires in vehicles. The fires resulted in 740 deaths. 'There were 99,500 incendiary and suspicious fires in structures reported to fire departments in 1988. The largest number of arson and suspected arson fires and losses occurred in residential properties.'[17] In 1988, juveniles accounted for some 43 per cent of those arrested for arson and 63 per cent were under the age of 25. According to the FBI, 18 per cent of arson offences were said to be solved; the figure is comparable with clear-up rates for other property crime. Sentences for serious cases of arson appeared to be getting longer – a trend in common with the UK.

Canada

Bradford reports that in 1977 there were 811 fire-related deaths and a loss of some $600 million. He notes an increase in over 4,000 in more recent years in the absolute number of reported fires. Bradford comments on the problem of bringing arson cases to court and securing convictions.[18]

Europe and Scandinavia[19]

In *Holland*, the number of cases of arson rose from 106 in 1963 to 1,600 in 1980 and the figure is said to be rising. In *Germany*, arson fires increased from 2,131 in 1960 to 9,408 in 1982 to over 10,000 in 1983. By 1984 the position was said to be getting worse. In *France*, between the years 1972 and 1982 there was 119 per cent increase in 'public property arson fires' and a 143 per cent increase in 'private property arson fires'. In *Belgium*, 30 per cent of fires are caused by arson, and in Brussels some 60 per cent are said to be so caused. In *Austria*, 22 per cent of the total cost of fires is due to arson. In *Sweden*, it is estimated that between 25 and 30 per cent of total fire costs are caused by arson and that a third of fires of unknown cause are probably caused by arson. In *Norway*, the figure is between 30 and 40 per cent. In *Finland*, the figure is somewhere in the region of 18 per cent. The comparative scale of the problem can be seen graphically in Figure 3.5.

Main targets

According to figures collected in 1985 by members of the European Conference of Fire Protection Associations (CFPA Europe), although no buildings were immune from arson attack, schools, factories, warehouses, places of entertainment and construction sites seemed to predominate as targets.[20]

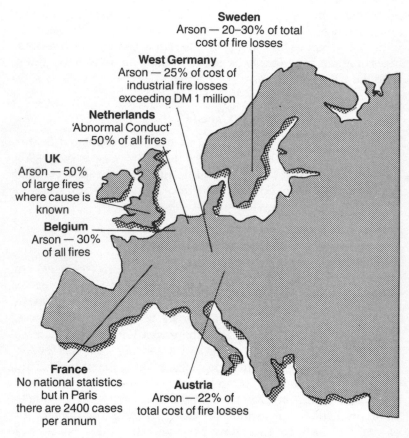

Sweden
Arson — 20–30% of total
cost of fire losses

West Germany
Arson — 25% of cost of
industrial fire losses
exceeding DM 1 million

Netherlands
'Abnormal Conduct'
— 50% of all fires

UK
Arson — 50%
of large fires
where cause is
known

Belgium
Arson — 30%
of all fires

France
No national statistics
but in Paris
there are 2400 cases
per annum

Austria
Arson — 22% of
total cost of fire losses

Figure 3.5 Arson – an international problem

Source: Home Office, *Report of the Working Group on the Prevention of Arson*, op. cit., p. 26. (Reproduced with permission.)

LEGAL ASPECTS

The law relating to arson would appear to have a lengthy history:

> Ancient Roman legal texts recognized arson and defined penalties for this offence. In France, prior to the French Revolution, deliberate arson was punished by death – hanging for commoners and decapitation for nobles . . . . Under some circumstances, arsonists were burned alive . . . . In Britain, during the reign of George II convicted arsonists . . . were banished from the country.[21]

Today, the legal expression of the offence of arson varies from one country to the next; no attempt is made to define it here other than in the UK. Other jurisdictions have comparable statutes and penalties. The word 'arson' itself is derived from Anglo and old French and from mediæval Latin: *ardere – ars* to burn (*Concise Oxford English Dictionary*). In England and Wales, prior to 1971, the offence of arson was dealt with under the Common Law. Currently, it is dealt with under the provisions of the Criminal Damage Act, 1971. Similar provisions apply in Northern Ireland. In Scotland, it is dealt with under a number of Common Law offences such as 'wilful fire-raising' and 'culpable and reckless fire-raising'. Section 1 of the Criminal Damage Act, 1971, states as follows:

(1) A person who without lawful excuse destroys or damages any property belonging to another intending to destroy or damage any such property or being reckless as to whether any such property would be destroyed or damaged shall be guilty of an offence.

(2) A person who without lawful excuse destroys or damages any property, whether belonging to himself or another -

    (a) intending to destroy or damage any property or being reckless as to whether any such property would be destroyed or damaged; and

    (b) intending by the destruction or damage to endanger the life of another or being reckless as to whether the life of another would be thereby endangered;

shall be guilty of an offence.

(3) An offence committed under this section by destroying or damaging property by fire *shall be charged as arson* [italics added].

Under Section 4 of the Act, the offences of both arson and endangering life are punishable with maximum penalties of life imprisonment.

It is of interest to note that the Law Commission, in its report (No. 29) that led to the introduction of the Criminal Damage Act, 1971, mentioned that 'one of the reasons for treating damage by fire differently from other types of damage was that many arsonists [were] mentally unbalanced and in need of treatment. Accordingly, the retention of arson with the maximum life penalty would help to ensure that such defendants could receive restriction orders' (under mental health legislation).[22]

CONCLUSION

The intention of this chapter has been to demonstrate that fire-raising, whether defined in legal or fire-service terms, is a widespread form of behaviour that has very grave consequences. Moreover, all the available evidence suggests (even if we allow for international variations in data collection and presentation) that it is increasing steadily. The data also suggest that it is not an easy offence to detect. Therefore, as great skill is required in its investigation, a short account of investigative methods is given in the next chapter.

4

THE INVESTIGATION OF
FIRE-RAISING

'When we have to tell what we have seen and found, it is our
business to give a true account, disguising nothing and keeping
nothing back. But let us be careful not to speak as if our little
plummets had sounded the depth of the universe'

Professor L.C. Miall

INTRODUCTION

The layperson's knowledge of forensic science investigation,
whether it be the work carried out by forensic scientists or by
forensic pathologists, most likely will have been gained from the
somewhat glamorised accounts provided in crime novels, plays
and on television. Popular forensic science heroes such as
'Quincey' will be familiar to television viewers on both sides of the
Atlantic; in the UK, those of an older generation will recall many
years ago Marius Goring's portrayal of *The Expert*. More recently,
the semi-documentary drama series *London's Burning* will have
brought fire detection and fire-fighting into the living rooms of
many. A number of recent documentaries concerning mis-
carriages of justice have also highlighted the very considerable
importance of forensic science work. All these depictions have
value if they provide insights, albeit small ones, into the activities
of forensic scientists. However, by their very nature, such attempts
to appeal to mass readers or audiences cannot depict adequately
the painstaking and often unsung efforts of those involved in
gathering and fitting together the pieces of a forensic science
puzzle. Moreover, as I show in Chapter 7, there are dangers in
over-glamorising fire, fire detection and fire-fighting, particularly
where children and young persons are concerned.

In this chapter I attempt to describe some aspects of fire investigation briefly, simply and in 'lay' fashion. Those wishing to pursue the topic in more depth could do no better than consult Cooke and Ide's *Principles of Fire Investigation*, the standard UK work.[1]

The basic general observational skills required in the investigation of fires have been described succinctly by a very experienced senior Home Office fire officer as follows:

> The major single element in establishing the cause of any fire is to discern its point of origin – the precise place where it started. To do this we need to examine the pattern of fire damage, the way in which it has spread three-dimensionally, commensurate with the known facts, with the situation before the fire, the material stored in the premises or the type of contents, their position in the building and the materials used in the construction of the building itself. The experienced fire-fighting officer . . . will . . . record such items as the colour and pressure of the smoke, the intensity and colour of the flames, the shape of the structure, the pattern of its collapse, particular smells and noises and the position and state of windows and doors etc. so that when the fire has been extinguished, either he on his own, or in conjunction with a more specially trained colleague, will attempt to ascertain the cause of the fire.[2]

BASIC INVESTIGATION

The initial steps to be taken in fire investigation are described in some detail in Chapter 5 of *The Arson Dossier* – a useful source of information produced by the Fire Protection Association.[3] As a first step, a form will be completed by an officer of the fire brigade in attendance at the scene. This will record cases thought to be of malicious or doubtful origin.[4] If the officers dealing with the fire 'on the spot' are doubtful about its cause or if there are fatalities involved, more specialist fire-service investigators may be called in to assist. If arson is suspected, the police will also be involved and a 'scene of crime' officer will normally be asked to attend. If necessary, and following discussion, the CID may also be called in. All such work obviously requires close and harmonious discussion and liaison at all stages of the investigation. The police

28

are provided with unambiguous guidelines in this respect in Home Office Circular 106/92.[5] In paragraphs 1–7, the steps that must be taken concerning liaison with the fire service are spelled out in some detail. More specific matters concerning detection and forensic investigation are dealt with in paragraphs 8–10, as follows:

(8) the senior fire officer and the police investigating officer will be aware of the potential contribution which the forensic science service can make to a fire investigation. It is the responsibility of the police investigating officer, in consultation with the scene of crime officer, to determine whether a forensic scientist should attend the scene;

(9) the Forensic Science Service is now an Agency of the Home Office. Its fire investigation services are available to the police and other investigating agencies, such as fire brigades. Its staff are available to attend fire scenes if requested to do so and to analyse fire debris for the presence of accelerants. It is particularly important for forensic scientists to attend scenes when it is anticipated that a prosecution may result from the investigation;

(10) the vital importance of scene preservation and/or the collection of evidence for subsequent scientific/technical investigation by the forensic science service cannot be over-emphasised.

Paragraphs 11 and 12 stress the need for full liaison and collaboration. The need to preserve materials that are found 'in situ' for further investigation is stressed throughout the circular instruction. I now turn to this more detailed further investigation; in this I draw heavily upon the work of Cooke and Ide, referred to above.

THE METHODS OF THE FORENSIC SCIENTIST

The Forensic Science Service in the UK exists to assist courts and the police with the investigation of crime. Fire investigation forms a highly specialised part of such a service and employs ever-developing sophisticated investigative techniques. Although predominantly laboratory based, forensic scientists are in attendance regularly at scenes of fires. They also provide training for fire-service staff in the early steps of investigation and identification of relevant information. Although a forensic scientist investigating fires will bring all his or her objectivity and scientific skills to bear upon the problem, he or she will not forget the very human element involved in the effects of fire on its victims; effects that are often tragic. Indeed, such awareness will no doubt spur the scientist on to sharpen his/her skills, particularly in those cases where serious fraud or foul play is suspected. He or she will also be conscious of the possible traumatic effects of incidents on those who are first on the scene – for example, the police and basic-grade fire officers. Such staff may well suffer from post-traumatic stress disorder – a syndrome acknowledged increasingly in both psychiatry and law. The tragic effects of fire are encapsulated in poignant fashion in a few lines by the late Charles Clisby – a very experienced fire officer:

> A child cries loudly in the night, its mother sharply coughs,
> For death has made an early start, at kind and creed it scoffs.
> Lost race against a ticking clock to infant's cot is run,
> Loved one is gathered up, the last maternal act is done.
> The infant and its mother soon unconscious of their doom,
> Await the gasping firemen in a corner of the room.[6]

It is perhaps worth pointing out here that Woodward has suggested more could be done by the senior managements of premises to make their own preliminary 'investigations of all fires; reporting any suspicious outbreaks to the authorities'.[7] He also asserts in the same paper that fire investigation training could well be longer and more intensive and that the Fire Protection Association, in conjunction with the various authorities involved, is actively promoting a greater consciousness of this need.

Some preliminary pointers

Macdonald suggests that there are some comparatively simple pointers that may give indications of malicious ignition or arson.[8] He cites, for example, the odour of specific combustible or flammable liquids, suggesting that these can sometimes be detected by an experienced fire officer at the scene of a fire. It is possible, however, to mistake paraffin for petrol and to make similar errors in initial detection. In addition, witnesses may have seen a person or persons running away from the scene. Experienced fire officers may spot the same spectator at more than one fire; such an individual may also show signs of singed clothing or hair. Macdonald (and others) have also suggested that a fully clothed person seen in the proximity of a fire in the early hours should arouse suspicion. If they have a camera with them it should arouse even more suspicion. The normal expectation would be for those closely involved to be in night attire. The excitement and arousal of the so-called compulsive fire-raiser at the scene may be evident in a flushed appearance or perhaps involuntary urination. Macdonald also lists some other useful pointers, such as trails of inflammable liquids and signs of forced entry. The removal of valuable items from the scene of the fire might be suggestive of arson, as it may indicate theft or preservation of property by the owner. Ide (personal communication, December 1992) suggests that very few fire-raisers willingly endanger pets; although they might set fire to a house recklessly endangering neighbours' and firemen's lives, they would normally put the cat out and even remove a bird cage and goldfish bowl before starting the fire. Indications of vandalism prior to a fire, or the presence of many live and spent matches, may be highly suggestive of juvenile fire-raising; the piling up of a house-owner's prized possessions in the middle of the site of a conflagration may be indicative of a fire motivated by revenge on the part of the rejected partner. Those whose fire-raising is motivated by financial gain may well construct elaborate alibis for their whereabouts at the time of the fire. Cooke and Ide add other items to those cited by Macdonald: for example, repeated or numerous fires; 'booby-trapping' or other tactics used to prevent access by fire-fighters; interference with sprinkler systems and other fire-fighting devices; specific targets (such as premises belonging to ethnic or other minority groups); destruction of specific records or similar data.

Other, more specific factors

Cooke and Ide list a number of additional and more specific factors. These are: multiple fire locations; unusual disposition of the contents of premises; presence of incendiary materials; the unusually rapid spread of fire; the fact that the value of the stock of a shop or warehouse does not appear to match the subsequent claims to insurance companies; evidence of a further crime (e.g.

homicide); obstructive behaviour towards investigating officers by the owner of the premises. They list forty-four possible reasons for suspicion but, as they wisely state, 'they must be regarded as reasons for suspicion only and do not in themselves provide absolute proof of deliberate action.'[9]

Cooke and Ide enumerate a number of other important steps to be taken in the more *detailed* investigation of fires. They stress the need to preserve items that may later prove to be useful, as, for example, when fraud is suspected. Items of particular interest for subsequent analysis may include the following:

1 Debris or clothing that may require to be tested for the presence of flammable liquids.
2 Domestic and industrial appliances which need to be examined for evidence of misuse or malfunction.
3 The collection of materials that can be used for burning tests to determine, for example, the ease with which they can be ignited or how speedily flames will spread across their surfaces.

Cooke and Ide advise extreme care in the actual removal of items from the scene so that contamination may be avoided, thus facilitating subsequent more sophisticated laboratory tests. Similar care should be exercised in the removal and preservation of appliances thought to be defective. The authors stress throughout the need for the utmost attention to detail. Forensic science investigation is not a field of en- deavour for the sloppy-minded or the heavy-handed. In recent years, fire investigation has become increasingly sophisticated in the UK, Europe, the USA and Japan; it has been greatly facilitated by the introduction of computer science and technology.

Arson and murder

Cooke and Ide suggest that 'Fire is such a good destroyer of evidence that numerous cases of arson associated with murder have probably been missed.'[10] They indicate some questions that can be usefully addressed in order to facilitate detection of this association:

(a) Can the victim be identified?
(b) Was the victim dead when the fire started?
(c) Is there evidence to show that the fire was deliberately started?

(d) If so, was it started with the intention of destroying evidence connected with the body?

(e) Is there any physical evidence remaining which can indicate how the victim died?

(f) Is there any evidence at the scene which can indicate who committed the offence?[11]

TRAINING FOR FIRE INVESTIGATION

The training of full-time fire investigators is highly specialised and time-consuming. As with training in other highly technical and professional fields, it should never end. The best forms of training will attempt to bring together practice and theory through the use of careful observation by the trainee of more experienced officers at work 'on site' and by theory taught in the lecture room and the laboratory. The *Arson Dossier*, already referred to, includes, in summary form, a statement of twelve essential components of a typical basic course in fire investigation. The suggestions for such a course allow for variation according to local need:

1 The role of the various parties involved in fire investigation.
2 Sources of information (for example, the development of interviewing skills, making sketches, plans, use of photography and other specialist techniques).
3 Fire science (basic chemistry, physics, the nature of explosives).
4 Fire Protection Devices (fire detectors and sprinklers).
5 The reaction of materials to fire.
6 Electricity as a source of fire.
7 Technology of fire investigation.
8 Investigation of 'fatal' fires.
9 Techniques of laboratory analysis.
10 Problems associated with special sites (for example, vehicles, trains, aircraft, ships).
11 Legal aspects (relevant legislation, the role of the expert witness, the giving of oral evidence).
12 'Hands-on' experience – fire fighting, use of case studies.[12]

CONCLUSION

The investigation of the cause of fires is a difficult and painstaking undertaking, particularly in the case of those fires that are thought to be of malicious origin. It requires a very high degree of alertness, shrewd observation, scientific skill and a capacity for good liaison work. Such qualities, exercised promptly, may provide significant early clues to the activities *and motives* of those who raise fires unlawfully. I consider these in some detail in the next two chapters.

5

ADULT FIRE-RAISERS: MOTIVES AND MANAGEMENT

'A little fire is quickly trodden out,
Which being suffered rivers cannot quench.'
Henry VI, Pt 3, Act IV, Scene viii

'Heat not a furnace for your foe so that
it singe yourself.'
Henry VIII, Act I, Scene i

'Can a man take fire to his bosom and
his clothes not be burned?'
Proverbs 6: 27

A CAUTIONARY NOTE

It should have become obvious from the preceding chapters that people set fires for reasons that are often complex and ill-understood. Sometimes, as we shall see, such persons may be adjudged to have been motivated by a degree of mental disorder. However, as I and many others have indicated elsewhere, the precise relationship between mental disorder and criminality is by no means as clear-cut as some would think. Some people's 'madness' may appear to be closely associated with their criminal behaviour; in other cases the association is less clear; in yet others it would appear that a person can be both 'mad' and 'bad'.[1] The case of Daniel McNaghten illustrates this point. McNaghten tried to shoot Robert Peel, the British Prime Minister; in fact, he shot and fatally injured Peel's Secretary, Drummond. At his trial, evidence was given that McNaghten was suffering from what would be described today as paranoid delusions, believing that he was the subject of a Tory conspiracy. For many years it has

35

been widely held that McNaghten's illness was the sole explanation of his behaviour. It is now believed, by some, that McNaghten may have been in fact involved with a political sect actively engaged in activities against the Tories.

Despite the need for caution that such examples demonstrate, it is often helpful, when trying to understand deviant and criminal behaviour, to try to attempt to classify it and to construct typologies that may enhance our attempts at management. At least it should serve to provide a starting point for further work. With this in mind, two colleagues and I tried some years ago to put together a fairly simple classification of imprisoned arsonists. This had as its main aim a description of their motivations.[2] However, not surprisingly, we found ourselves in difficulties, because parts of this classification dealt with motivation quite adequately, but other parts were merely descriptive of disordered mental states that may or may not have determined motives. In addition, sometimes the motivation was unclear or, as I shall show later, more than one motive may have been involved. In a recent contribution, Soothill has gone so far as to indicate that such attempts may even be unhelpful since they attempt to do too much. He states that they 'are not an aid to understanding "arson", even less arsonists, but are much closer to being a scheme for knowing where to file the instances of arson which may come to the attention of psychiatrists'.[3] He also suggests, not without *some* justification, that

> it is a dangerous practice to collapse very different categories of explanation within one general classification. In essence, there is a need to distinguish between different instances of arson, on the one hand, and the characteristics of arsonists (including motives) on the other.[4]

A similar point is made by Wooden and Berkey in writing about children who raise fires (see also Chapter 6). They suggest that it is necessary to distinguish between behavioural characteristics of fire-raisers, various types of fire-raisers *and* their motives.[5] In the study of imprisoned arsonists referred to earlier, we considered that it would be desirable for a psychiatric opinion to be obtained on all arsonists, because the motivation was often very complex. This view finds some support in the *Report of the Working Group on the Prevention of Arson*. The Working Group note the view of the Court of Appeal that 'a psychiatric report should *normally* be sought in cases of arson'.[6] This is a view also supported by Macdonald, who states that 'all persons charged with arson should undergo psychiatric examination'.[7] Soothill is less favourably inclined to psychiatric intervention:

> Perhaps because of the importance of the crime and because of the puzzle of explanation, psychiatry has had a long history of being interested in the offence. Sadly, the link with psychiatry has not always contributed a fuller understanding of the activity.[8]

In summary, it would appear that in cases other than those where the motivation is *abundantly clear and non-pathological*, a psychiatric opinion can be valuable. However, Soothill is right in alerting us to the dangers of expecting psychiatrists to provide answers to near insoluble problems and of adding to the tendency to 'psychiatrise' delinquency. It is also very important to stress yet again the importance of mixed motives for this very serious crime. Their importance is stressed by a non-psychiatric professional – the crime writer Ruth Rendell: 'To wreak death might have been the primary motive, but the lust for spoliation was there as well. It gilded the lily.'[9] As a general introduction to the classification that follows, readers may find Figure 5.1 helpful in its depiction of the main motives of arsonists, the situations in which they may carry out their activities and their main targets.

CLASSIFICATION AND MOTIVATION

Bearing in mind the reservations and deficiencies expressed above, I propose to give a selection of attempts to classify motives for arson and then to provide illustrative case material for each main group. Inciardi suggests the following typology: (a) revenge; (b) excitement fire-setting; (c) institutionalised fire-setters; (d) insurance claim fire-setters; (e) arson to cover up another crime.[10] This has all the dangers of the mixed classification complained about by Soothill. More recently, Ravataheino, in a Finnish study of 180 arsonists arrested in Helsinki, classified his subjects under the following headings: (1) insurance fraud; (2) revenge, jealousy, hatred, envy, grudge; (3) sensation; (4) alcoholic and mental patients, and the 'temporarily disturbed'; (5) vandalism; (6) pyromaniacs; (7) children under 15.[11] This classification is more finely nuanced but still suffers from being a mixture of motives

MOTIVE	TYPE	TYPICAL ARSONIST	MAJOR TARGETS	PROBABLE FREQUENCY
Vandalism	Deliberate	Male teenager	Any but particularly schools and public buildings	High
Playing with fire	—	Child under 10 years old	Dwellings Schools Rubbish skips	High
Crime concealment	(a) Vehicle crime	Young males 15–25 years old	Cars	Moderate
	(b) Other crime	Various offenders	Any	Moderate
Revenge	(a) Domestic	Any	Dwellings	Moderate
	(b) Non-domestic		Any	
Fraud	(a) Insurance fraud	Insurance policyholder		
	(b) Avoiding planning restrictions	Property owner or person acting on his behalf	Business premises	Moderate
Political	(a) Terrorist	Member of political organisation or movement	Retail and other high public profile premises	Low
	(b) Protestor			
	(c) Racist	Insufficient information	Ethnic minority businesses and homes	
	(d) Riot	Usually young males	Inner city buildings	
Mental illness*	—	Any	Any	Low

* This does not include a significant number of people who can be described as acting under emotional pressure as opposed to being diagnosed as mentally ill.

Figure 5.1 Motives for arson: the arson matrix

Source: Home Office, Standing Conference on Crime Prevention: *Report of the Working Group on the Prevention of Arson*, London, December 6, 1988, p. 13. (Reproduced with permission.)

and characteristics. Faulk provides two useful broad groupings: Group I consists of those cases in which the fire serves as a means to an end (such as revenge, fraud or a plea for help); Group II consists of those cases where the *fire itself* is the phenomenon of interest.[12] On the basis of the study of imprisoned arsonists referred to earlier we suggested the following classification:

1 Arson committed for financial reward.
2 Arson committed to cover up another crime.
3 Arson committed for political purposes (for example, for specific terrorist or similar activities).
4 Self-immolation as a political gesture.
5 Arson committed for mixed motives (for example, in a state of minor depression [reactive], as a cry for help, or under the influence of alcohol).
6 Arson due to the presence of an actual mental or associated disorder.
   (a) Severe affective disorder.
   (b) Schizophrenia.
   (c) 'Organic' disorders (for example, brain tumour, injury, temporal lobe epilepsy, dementing processes, disturbed metabolic processes).
   (d) Mental subnormality (retardation), impairment.
7 Arson due to motives of revenge:
   (a) against an individual or individuals (specific).
   (b) against society or others more generally.
8 Arson committed as an attention-seeking act (but excluding motives set out under [5] above), and arson committed as a means of deriving sexual satisfaction/excitement. (Pyromania.)
9 Arson committed by young adults (16 and over). (Vandalism.)
10 Arson committed by children. (See Chapter 6.)[13]

Again, the weaknesses of this classification are also apparent. In the *Report of the Working Group on the Prevention of Arson* a study was undertaken of 238 offenders involved in 214 detected incidents of arson in England and Wales, based upon probation officers' social inquiry reports and supplemented by material in the case files of social services departments. The analysis indicated that some 50 per cent were due to an 'emotional mental state' (this was not defined further, but 8 per cent were diagnosed formally as mentally ill); 3 per cent were due to concealment of crime; 4.2 per cent to individual vandalism; 14 per cent to group vandalism; 7 per cent to disputes; and 21.3 per cent to revenge. There was an obvious overlap between arson regarded as attributable to dispute and that adjudged to be motivated by revenge. For example, 'when arson occurred following a dispute between individuals it was only regarded as revenge when a period of time had elapsed and evidence of planned rather than impulsive retaliation emerged.'[14] A useful and practical classification is provided by Cooke and Ide. They suggest ten groupings, but in so doing they also wisely emphasise a degree of overlap:

1 Insurance fraud fires, ignited by the insured.
2 Ditto, ignited by a hired 'torch'.
3 Fires started by business rivals.
4 Fires started by employees.
5 Fires started by political activists.
6 Fires to conceal other crimes.
7 Fires started by children.
8 Fires started by vandals.
9 Fires started by attention-seekers and enthusiasts.
10 Fires started by mentally deranged fire-setters.[15]

SOME GENERAL CHARACTERISTICS

Before proceeding to consider motivation in more detail by way of illustrative case material,[16] it may be useful to summarise briefly a few general characteristics of arsonists. They are mostly young adult males, many of whom have serious relationship problems, both at the general and the sexual level. A large proportion have problems with alcohol and many are not very bright. When women commit repeated acts of arson or have a history of mental disorder, they are more likely than their male counterparts to be given psychiatric as compared to penal disposals. One can discern an interesting change in the incidence of females as fire-raisers. As indicated in Chapter 2, in the nineteenth century arson was seen to be the prerogative of frustrated teenage female servants. There then followed a marked diminution in that incidence. This was followed by a gradual increase in the representation of women amongst arsonists. This might be accounted for by the increasing representation of women involved in general crimes of violence and participation in terrorist activities. Some workers have found evidence of unstable childhoods and serious psychological disturbance for both groups. A direct sexual motivation for the commission of arson is *not* a frequent occurrence, but its relevance will be considered when I deal with pyromania. In general, reconviction for further arson is not high overall, but when followed up for long periods a number of arsonists who commit the offence for vengeful purposes tend to repeat it.[17]

STEPS TOWARDS UNDERSTANDING

'I stand as if a mine beneath my feet,
Were ready to be blown up.'
The Duchess of Malfi,
Act III, Scene ii

Whatever the imperfections of the attempts at classification provided above, I propose to use an amalgam of them to consider explanations and motives in more detail; and to illustrate these, where possible, with case vignettes. Fire-raising by children – as distinct from young adults – is considered separately in Chapter 6.

Arson committed for financial or other reward

In these cases, 'the property burned can vary considerably in value from industrial premises costing millions of pounds, through domestic premises and cars, down to single items of furniture or articles of clothing.'[18] The apparent increase in the offence of burning vehicles referred to in Chapter 3 would fall into this category if, for example, the objective was to avoid hire-purchase payments or to seek some kind of compensation from an insurance company. However, the motives may not be so clear-cut, as some individuals who raise fires for apparent gain in this fashion may, for example, also be suffering from a degree of depression, due to overwhelming financial burdens or the effects of the recession. Rix, who has recently studied a group of 70 arsonists in the north of England, discovered that arson as an attempt to be rehoused represented a quite frequent motive.[19]

Vignette 1

A husband who set fire to the two-roomed 'mice ridden flat' where he lived with his wife and children was given an eighteen-month suspended sentence of imprisonment coupled with a supervision order. The local housing authority had provided numerous mouse traps but had declined to rehouse the family. The defendant set fire to the flat having made sure his family and other residents were outside. The judge expressed his sympathy for the man and his family, having heard that their living conditions were 'appalling' (*The Independent*, August 4, 1990, p. 3).

Vignette 2

A man said to be dying of cancer embarked on a career of arson and blackmail in an effort to secure funds to provide for his wife. He had planted a series of home-made explosive devices in a group of German supermarkets. These consisted of materials such as weedkiller, sugar and matchheads. No one was hurt, but damage amounting to some £100,000 was caused. Having set the devices he phoned the companies demanding money. He was jailed for two and a half years (*The Independent*, March 24, 1990, p. 4).

Sometimes arson committed for a degree of financial reward can have tragic consequences, as the following case illustrates.

Vignette 3

A woman set fire to her one-bedroomed flat causing the destruction not only of her own home but of two neighbouring flats as well. As a result of the fires, an elderly neighbour, who lived two flats away, sustained injuries from which he died. In court it was alleged that the defendant had doubled her insurance on her home contents and set the fire in order to deal with increasing debts. It was also alleged that, on the night before the fire, she had removed some of her property to a relative's home. (See the remarks on fire detection in Chapter 4.) The judge told the defendant that although she did not intend to cause injury she knew there were elderly residents nearby and that the risk of injury would be high. She was sentenced to seven years' imprisonment (*The Independent*, June 16, p. 5, and June 30, 1992, p. 5).

Cooke and Ide identify, under my first category, two further forms of arson for gain. The first is the use of what the Americans describe as a hired 'torch', or professional arsonist. They suggest that the standards of performance by such offenders vary considerably – from great sophistication to bungling amateurism.[20] The second are fires started by business rivals. Such fires have much in common with insurance fraud fires. Cooke and Ide suggest that

> The main differences are that the fire-damaged business is likely to have been thriving, otherwise it will not have seemed a threat to the rival concern, and the fire raiser is not likely to have spent so much time in the building setting up the fire. In addition it is possible that the fire-damaged premises may not be adequately insured.[21]

Arson to conceal other crimes

Sometimes acts of arson will be committed in order to conceal a variety of offences. These may range from theft to murder. In respect of the latter, readers will recall the need to investigate fire fatalities with particular care, referred to in Chapter 4. Some fires will cause enormous damage, particularly if they are set to cover offences such as theft in large and well-stocked warehouses. Woodward cites two instances of this kind of fire-raising.[22] In the first, a warehouse of a shipping company was destroyed by fire. The goods stored there included TV sets, car tyres and other easily combustible items. From the forensic examination at the scene of the fire it was apparent that theft had taken place before the fire had been raised. In the second case he cites a fire raised in a bonded warehouse containing video recorders, amongst other items. The warehouse had been the object of repeated pilfering in the preceding months and it was considered that the fire had been raised deliberately to divert attention away from these thefts.

Arson committed for political purposes

There are two main motives for arson committed by political activists. The first concerns the desire to destroy the property of those they hold a grudge against; the second is the publicity gained for the activists' cause. The alleged destruction of 'second homes' by Welsh activists would be illustrative of the first, and the work of the IRA and other paramilitary and fascist organisations would be illustrative of the second. A most disturbing trend in the last year has been numerous outbreaks of arson and similar attacks on so-called 'foreigners' in Germany. I have before me as this chapter is being drafted a graphic and sinister account of such activity in the north-western German town of Möllen:

> Two young girls and a woman, all of them Turkish, died from burns after their house . . . was fire-bombed . . . . Neighbours spoke of screaming and crying from inside the house where the three died, as it was rapidly consumed by flames. Nine people were seriously injured, including one child, both of whose legs were broken by jumping from an upper story window.

An elderly, physically handicapped next-door neighbour said

> I cannot get the sight of her body out of my mind. Little Yeliz was just a charred bundle when the firemen covered her up on the stretcher. The stairs must have been soaked with petrol for the whole thing just went up like a bonfire.

The Federal State Prosecutor said that the use of the words 'Heil Hitler' in an anonymous phone call 'indicates that the perpetrators wanted to help restore a Nazi dictatorship in Germany' (*The Independent*, November 24, 1992, pp. 1 and 10).

Although the main motives are often seen to be political, there are also sometimes psycho-pathological elements, such as the feeling of power such activities may provide. To this extent, the motivation may be mixed as, for example, in the case of other offences such as serious sexual assault.

Vignette 4

The activities of the Welsh extremists are well known in respect of the first motive identified above. A recent report in the national

44

press indicated that

> Fears that the long-running arson campaign by Welsh
> extremists . . . against English owned property in Wales is
> entering a new phase were raised after fire-raising attacks
> over the weekend. Potentially the most serious was the
> planting of an incendiary bomb at government offices in
> Carmarthen yesterday. Police called in a bomb disposal
> team and the device was defused. A house near Pwllheli,
> Gwynedd, owned by Wolverhampton social services
> department was badly damaged in another attack. An
> empty second home outside Bala, Gwynedd, was burnt and
> a similar property near Tywyn, Gwynedd, was gutted.
>
> *(The Independent,* November 2, 1992, p. 3,
> and November 10, 1992, p. 1)

The more extreme work of animal rights activists is of course
well-known for the ferocity of its attacks on those they believe to
be the enemy. The Animal Liberation Front has carried out
serious attacks over the years. In an article in *The Independent
Magazine* of October 31, 1992, there is an interesting pen-portrait
of Ronnie Lee, who has been serving a sentence of ten years'
imprisonment for 'conspiring with and inciting others to commit
damage in department stores that sold furs' – a charge that he has
always denied (p. 50). However, he has 'never repudiated the
ALF's tactic of "economic sabotage"' (p. 50). Like many others of
his views, Mr Lee holds very powerful beliefs as to the justice of
his cause. Such zealousness may of course blind such people to
the damage they may cause others. Upon receiving his sentence
Lee is said to have told Lord Justice Lawton, 'That's all right'.
'Even so,' the article continues, 'Lee is genuinely offended that
Lawton should have presided over his fate. "People who eat meat
and don't give a fuck about animals have no right to sit in
judgement over vegetarians who are trying to save animals"' (p.
53). Presumably he might have been happier to have been
sentenced by a vegetarian or vegan judge.

Sometimes the cause of these and similar attacks is hard to
discern. Christian Wolmar in *The Independent* of April 29, 1991 (p.
7), reports that a spate of fires in a Hampshire hamlet has baffled
detectives. He describes

13 fires or arson attempts in the past three years in this hamlet of 20 houses whose only communal facility is a post box . . . . Of the five thatched houses, two have been attacked twice, and two once. 'At first, it was thought the fires were a series of coincidences, but now there is no doubt an arsonist is at work.'

Finally, a rather unusual illustration from the USA:

Vignette 5

Woodward reports upon a Boston

seven-member arson ring, comprising police and fire-fighters : . . formed to protest against the state tax-cutting measures, which would involve a loss of jobs. . . . During a period of two years they were involved in setting 269 fires expertly, in which at least 282 people were injured . . . . It was only due to a demonstration of over-exuberance during a fire that one of the ring was caught.[23]

Cases of self-immolation

'And lifting up a fearful eye to view what fire was near'
Robert Southwell, 'The Burning Babe'

These cannot be regarded as cases of arson in the true sense of the term, but an act of self-immolation may have serious consequences for the lives of others, as the following vignette shows.

Vignette 6

This concerned the case of a young woman in the north of England who tried to kill herself in her bedroom by dousing her body in petrol and then attempting to ignite it. This having failed, she subsequently tried to blow herself up (and the other residents of the house) by turning on the gas taps and striking matches. Fortunately, this attempt also failed. However, the legal ingredients of a charge of endangering life through arson were sustainable and the defendant was admitted to a psychiatric hospital under a court order. At the time she was found to have been suffering from a serious depressive illness, but subsequently made a good recovery. This case also demonstrates the problems of trying to 'pigeon hole' people since the young woman's problem could have been classified under the heading of mental disorder – to be dealt with later.

We read not infrequently of 'outbreaks' of ritualised self-destruction – mainly for political reasons. A report in *The Independent* of May 21, 1991 (p. 2), describes the ritual suicide of Kim Ki Sol, who wrote 'There are many meanings to my act today' before 'setting himself alight and jumping in flames from the roof of a seven storey building at Seoul's Sogang University'. In both North and South Korea and elsewhere a disturbing increase in such behaviour has been noted. Cult self-immolation is not of course a new phenomenon. Reference has already been made in Chapter 2 to the ritual of *Suttee*. Barker describes a number of young members of a group known as Ananda Marga, 'who immolated themselves' as a protest 'against the imprisonment in India of their leader'. Two of them said that their 'self-immolation [was] done [as the result of a] personal and independent decision. It [was] out of love for all human beings, for the poor, for the exploited, the suffering.'[24] Topp has drawn attention to the extent to which self-destruction by fire seems to have shown a slow but steady increase in penal establishments in recent years.[25] He has suggested that such individuals who choose an obviously very painful method of death are likely to be those who have some capacity for divorcing their feelings from their consciousness. Some may be epileptics in a disturbed state of consciousness. (One such case has been described in some detail by Newton.)[26] However, in all such cases of self-immolation, we should remember that people probably vary enormously in their pain thresholds. Some would succumb very quickly to such an agonising method of self-destruction. One imagines that shock and asphyxiation would probably occur within a very short space of time so that the severe pain caused by the burning of vital tissues would not have to be endured for too long. Such may have been the fate of some of the early martyrs who chose to suffer death at the stake. Occasionally, such sufferers were 'granted the merciful privilege . . . of having a small bag of gunpowder hung around [the] neck in order to speed their demise and so reduce [their] suffering'.[27]

Arson committed for mixed and unclear reasons

I have already indicated how difficult it is to ascribe a single motive for a crime like arson; more often than not the motives appear to be mixed. In the sample of 113 imprisoned arsonists referred to earlier, my colleagues and I found a number of cases in which it was difficult to attribute a *single specific* motive. We were forced to try to subdivide the group – in the following way. First, we had a small number of cases in which the offender appeared to be suffering from a mild (reactive) degree of depressive illness at the time of the crime. Such depression is sometimes associated with anger directed at a spouse or partner, *so there may also be an element of revenge involved.* Second, there were cases in which the arson appeared to be a disguised plea for help. Third, one or two cases in which the arson appeared to have been precipitated by a sudden separation from a near relative or loved one or by a bereavement. Fourth, some cases in which alcohol seemed to play a part. As with other crimes, the ingestion of alcohol features quite significantly. The offender may state that he or she had been drinking very heavily at the time and cannot recall what happened. Such a lack of recall may be due, in rare cases, to genuine alcoholic amnesia, but is more likely to be due to a befuddled state caused by intoxication. It is possible that a fire may be set accidentally as a result of such a state. However, in my experience, such fires are comparatively rare. The degree of mixed motivation that occurs is well illustrated in the following vignette.

Vignette 7

This concerns a man in his mid-thirties with a history of personality disorder. He had a history of highly disturbed behaviour including setting fire to the parental home on one occasion and making numerous 'false alarm' calls to the police and fire brigade. Following a period of compulsory hospitalisation by a court for one of his fire-raising episodes, he had been discharged to a mental health after-care facility. He did not get on at all well with the staff and considered they were 'picking' on him. During a depressive episode in which he had been drinking heavily, he set fire to the establishment, causing damage amounting to several thousand pounds.

Arson due to serious mental disorder

Under this heading I consider the functional psychoses (the schizophrenias and manic-depressive illness), organic disorders, personality disorder and mental impairment. The revenge motive, which may sometimes be associated with mental disturbance and pyromania in its own right, is considered under a separate heading. It is important to emphasise yet again that the categories overlap and are not discrete.

Schizophreniform illness and arson

A number of arsonists, particularly those detained in the special hospitals or in secure units, suffer from a clearly diagnosable schizophrenic illness of one type or another.[28] Some of them have set fire to dwellings or other premises as a result of their delusional and/or hallucinatory experiences. One such offender/patient said to me 'I set fire to [the house] to get rid of the evil in it.' Others will allege that they have seen the image of God and heard Him directing them to raise fires. Sometimes the association is not quite so clear-cut, as the following vignette demonstrates.

Vignette 8

A man in his late forties, who was already detained in an ordinary psychiatric hospital in the west country for an offence of arson, attempted to set fire to his room with matches and clothing. A nurse spotted the small but growing blaze; it was put out, and the patient and others were not physically harmed. However, it was thought to be advisable to bring charges so that he could be held in more secure conditions. Accordingly, a hospital order was made in the crown court with added restrictions without limit of time. He had previous convictions for criminal damage and arson, on two occasions having been dealt with by means of hospital orders without restrictions. He had become ill as an adolescent and been diagnosed as suffering from schizophrenia and personality disorder. The latter had become more marked as time went by, probably, as is sometimes the case, as a result of the influence of his schizophrenic illness. He had become increasingly subject to hallucinations and delusions but it was difficult to determine the extent to which he acted directly as

49

a result of these in his fire-raising activities. In hospital, though he remained ill and was sometimes subject to delusions and hallucinations, he had responded to medication. It was hoped that at some future date it would be possible to place him in less secure conditions. He was thought to be not basically an arsonist, but a person whose illness led him sometimes to light fires.

Occasionally, sufferers from a chronic schizophrenic illness may become vagrants. In their wanderings about the countryside they *may* set fire to a building or themselves as a result of their impaired mental state. However, Virkunnen makes the important point that they do not often choose dwellings for such activities but smaller objects such as telegraph poles or fences.[29]

Severe affective disorder and arson

I have already shown in Vignette 7 how a mild degree of depressive disorder may contribute to an episode of fire-raising. I now consider the connection between more serious affective disorder and this behaviour.

Vignette 9

An inquest was told how a man in his forties doused his wife and two sons with petrol, then set fire to them believing that God had told him to do so. Fortunately his wife and two sons were saved by neighbours, but the man died from burns to most of his body. He is alleged to have said 'God told me to do this. He's been speaking to me for 20 years.' A psychiatrist told the inquest that the man had been suffering from a 'substantial depressive illness' and that he believed the 'family would be better off dead'. The coroner recorded a verdict that the man killed himself while the balance of his mind was disturbed. Had he survived, probably he would have been charged and, if successfully prosecuted, been made liable to a mental health disposal (*The Independent*, May 29, 1992, p. 5).

Vignette 10

Probably the most well-known example of a manic-depressive arsonist is that of Jonathan Martin, who set fire to York Minster in

1829. His story is described in some detail by Scott;[30] the following short account draws upon Scott's history of events. There is also an interesting painting of the effects of the fire housed in the archives of the Bethlem Royal Hospital; a black and white reproduction can be found as part of Soothill's chapter on arson already referred to.[31]

Martin was born in 1792, the third of five children. His background seems to have been somewhat disturbed and as a child he was given to wandering. While on naval service he was involved in putting out a serious fire on board ship. During this time he appears to have developed the notion that he had a special relationship with God and, according to his contemporaries, seems to have suffered from what we would describe as serious mood swings of a manic-depressive variety. He left the navy in 1810, married, and had one son. His preoccupation with religion continued and he became convinced that the Church lacked discipline. He became increasingly disturbed, much to the consternation of his wife and local people. He was 'certified' and committed to an asylum, but absconded on numerous occasions. He was eventually left at large in the community. With hindsight this was probably not a very wise course of action. He went to Lincoln and subsequently to York. His delusional ideas became increasingly grandiose and he sent angry letters to the clergy at the Minster. Eventually he went there and 'set fire to paper, music and books'. The blaze spread with devastating effect causing extensive damage. On remand in prison he remained alternatively depressed and manic. At his trial in 1829, on the basis of the medical evidence before the court, the jury found him not guilty by reason of insanity in only seven minutes. It is important to remember that in those days the offence he had committed was punishable by death. It is said that when the charge was put to him at the assize he replied 'It was not me my Lord, but my God did it. It is quite common for Him to punish to the third and fourth generation, and to show mercy to those that fear Him and keep His commandments.' He was committed to Bethlem, where he died in 1838. It is difficult to make a modern diagnosis on ancient retrospective evidence, but Scott's suggestion that he was probably a manic-depressive seems correct. At his trial he was described as suffering from 'monomania', a precursor of the term pyromania. Scott notes that Jonathan's son Richard killed himself in a state of depression some three months after his father's death.

He postulated that this may help to confirm the diagnosis of severe affective disorder.

Vignette 11

A young man in his thirties became increasingly grandiose in his ideas and demonstrated all the characteristic signs of hypomania. He was convinced that the computer firm he worked for was not active enough in promoting its sales. He developed all kinds of excessively ambitious and quite irrational schemes to improve matters and became hostile to any interference. His employers tolerated his behaviour for some time since they thought that his euphoria and far-fetched ideas were but an extension of his usual somewhat over-active and over-zealous manner. However, it gradually became apparent that he was ill and steps were taken to try to make him cease his activities and seek medical help. Being quite without insight (a key feature of this illness) he became angry at those he felt did not understand or appreciate him. In 'retaliation', he set fire to the salesroom, causing damage amounting to many thousands of pounds. He was charged with arson, brought to court, and made the subject of a hospital order with restrictions under the Mental Health Act. With medication his condition improved sufficiently for him to be discharged into the community under supervision.

Arson associated with 'organic' disorders

Very occasionally, arson may be committed by a person who is suffering from some form of 'organic' disorder (for example, brain tumour, injury, epilepsy, dementia and metabolic disturbances). For instance, epilepsy is not commonly associated with arson. However, it may be present in cases where the crime has been committed openly and in the presence of witnesses by someone who does not appear to be in a state of normal consciousness. Nevertheless, the epilepsy is more likely than not to be found to be associated with other adverse personal and social circumstances, notably poor family relationships. In their study of 50 arsonists detained in Grendon Underwood Psychiatric Prison, Hurley and Monahan found that 20 per cent had a history of head injury with loss of consciousness but without other neurological consequences.[32]

Carpenter and King have described an interesting case in which a man temporarily developed a personality change, psychosis *and epilepsy* after having had brain surgery for a subarachnoid haemorrhage. While affected by these problems he set fire to his house and it was considered by the authors that his fire-raising was directly related to an epileptic seizure. He was charged, hospitalised, informally made a good recovery and remained symptom-free after some three years.[33] The authors also comment on the role of alcohol in such cases. The patient was not a heavy drinker but accepted advice not to drink at all because of its possible harmful effects on his condition. A further case prompted by the one just referred to has been described by Byrne and Walsh. This concerned a woman who set fire to a shop – one of a series of fires raised by her. She was originally given a diagnosis of personality disorder, but careful observation and re-assessment by the use of electro-encephalographic examination revealed gross abnormalities consistent with an epileptic focus in the temporal lobe of her brain. She was placed on a drug regime to deal with her newly diagnosed condition, has apparently remained symptom-free and her fire-raising behaviour has ceased.[34]

Vignette 12

A man of 65 suddenly embarked upon a series of fire-raising episodes in his home. He had hitherto had an unblemished record, and was popular with both family and friends. The only possible note of concern was that his wife had detected a small but increasing degree of mild irritability and forgetfulness. He was duly charged and appeared in court. A perceptive probation officer persuaded the court to seek psychiatric and neurological reports. He was found to be showing signs of early dementia. The court made a probation order but he eventually needed full-time residential care.

Vignette 13

A woman in her late thirties had a long history of aggressive behaviour that always seemed to be associated with her menstrual cycle. She had appeared in court on many occasions for a variety of offences of violence. However, they were usually of a minor variety and had been dealt with by either fines or other non-custodial penalties. Her current court appearance concerned two charges of arson in the house of a female friend with whom she had had a disagreement over the repayment of a sum of money. Her current offences again seemed to coincide with severe menstrual tension; she was made the subject of a probation order with a requirement for medical oversight of her condition.

Arson and mental impairment

The use of the preferred legal description is meant to encompass those conditions also recognised at various times under the terms deficiency, retardation, handicap, subnormality. Not infrequently a degree of mental impairment in offenders is also associated with personality disorder so the two conditions are considered together.

A history of mental impairment seems to occur quite frequently in those persons who have committed arson on more than one occasion. McKerracher and Dacre studied one such group of arsonists detained in Rampton (Special) Hospital (which at the time of their survey catered almost exclusively for dangerous mentally impaired [subnormal] offender-patients). They considered that the arsonists were more emotionally unpredictable than other Rampton patients and displayed a wider range of psychiatric symptoms than did other residents.[35] Very often, mentally impaired arsonists suffer from a variety of social and other handicaps as well. The following vignettes illustrate some of these combined difficulties.

Vignette 14

This concerns a woman in her late twenties, formally diagnosed as mildly mentally subnormal (impaired) and personality disordered, who came from a highly disturbed background. Her parents had fought for years before finally divorcing. A number of her siblings had been before the courts on numerous occasions. Much of her behaviour was of the attention-seeking variety and over the years she had set fire to a number of establishments in which she had been detained. The offence for which she had received a sentence of life imprisonment (later made the subject of a 'transfer direction' to hospital) consisted of setting fire to bedding and furniture in a local hospital.[36] Had it not been for the prompt intervention of the nursing staff a serious tragedy might have occurred involving the deaths of many patients and staff. This case illustrates just how serious arson is as an offence.

Vignette 15

This is the case of a man aged 50, currently detained in a special hospital. He had suffered brain damage as a child which had resulted in quite severe mental impairment. From a very early age he had exhibited aggressive behaviour towards his own family and others – particularly towards children. His fire-raising activities had started early in life and these had been interspersed with sexual offences and crimes of violence. He *claimed* that the sight of fire excited him sexually. His problems were compounded by the fact that in his early forties he had developed a concurrent psychotic illness in which he heard voices telling him to raise fires. The incident which brought him before the court on the occasion which resulted in his admission to a special hospital was an attempt to burn down a local psychiatric hospital to which he had been admitted informally. Such a case, and the two that follow, illustrates clearly how hard it is to try to make 'neat' classifications. The link between sexual arousal and fire is explored later.

Vignette 16

This concerned a man in his late thirties diagnosed as suffering from mental impairment and a degree of personality disorder. He had set fire to a store-room containing highly flammable materials. The fire spread quickly to a building next door where a number of people were working. He had a long history of fire-raising activities and making hoax telephone calls to the police and fire services. He also suffered from concurrent physical disabilities – a severe speech impediment and a limp which greatly affected his self-esteem. His main interest in life was in raising fires and he was regarded as highly dangerous by the hospital authorities. When mental impairment is accompanied by severe physical disability or disfigurement it presents greater problems because the offender has to cope with two or more very real handicaps. In such cases, arson is often a way of drawing attention to oneself and one's plight.

Such attention-seeking behaviour may present other hazards too, as is illustrated in a case that achieved national notoriety.

Vignette 17

This concerns a young man who was a self-confessed homicidal arsonist – with a very real need to draw attention to himself. Aged about 20 at the time of his trial, he was said to be of low intelligence; he also suffered from cerebral palsy and was said to be epileptic. A sad assemblage of handicaps one might think. He was also said to have been vengeful. He was originally charged with, and convicted of, a very large number of fires and killings, but was cleared in the Court of Appeal of one of these fires in which eleven elderly men had died. In this latter case the Court of Appeal considered that his conviction was unsafe – the court giving as its main reason 'the unsatisfactory nature of the forensic evidence' (*The Times*, December 3, 1983). However, he was sent to a special hospital for ten other fires which killed fifteen people. His case, which was investigated for a year by *The Sunday Times'* 'Insight' team (*The Sunday Times*, March 14, 1982), highlights an important issue in relation to arson committed by those who may be of limited intelligence. There may be such an overwhelming desire to seek attention that false confessions may be made. As with other recent cases, it is most important for those suspected of such offences and who may be mentally impaired to be accompanied by an 'appropriate adult', as the law now requires.

Arson motivated by revenge

'To bottomless perdition there to dwell
In adamantine chains and penal fire.'
Paradise Lost I: 47

In considering the link between motives of revenge and arson it is important to reiterate the point made earlier, that it is hazardous to try to place behaviours uncritically in discrete categories. For example, the vengeful arsonist may show clear signs of an identifiable mental illness, may be mentally and/or physically impaired, as in Vignette 17 above, or may not be 'ill' at all in any formal psychiatric sense.

Because vengeful arsonists appear to constitute a large and

potentially very dangerous group, it is necessary to deal with them and their problems in some detail. However, before doing so, it may be helpful to develop some aspects of the historical perspective touched upon in Chapter 2. The historian Keith Thomas suggests that in the sixteenth and seventeenth centuries, perhaps next to the plague, fire was the greatest threat to life. For example, candles could cause havoc with thatched houses; fire precautions were primitive in workplaces, as were fire-fighting techniques. (There was no organised form of fire insurance until the 1690s.) There was also a firm belief that fire and other disasters were punishments for wrong-doing. Deliberate fire-raising was also a common form of revenge in the seventeenth century:

> for those who felt themselves injured by their neighbours, arson required no great physical strength or financial resources and could easily be concealed. It was an indiscriminate means of vengeance however, for a fire, once started, was likely to spread. As such, it perhaps appealed especially to those whose hatred for their neighbours was all-embracing.[37]

Thomas cites numerous cases of alleged witches threatening to or actually burning down the houses of neighbours or those they felt had wronged them. Sometimes charges of arson and sorcery overlapped. Thomas cites the case of Anne Foster, who was convicted at Northampton in 1674 of bewitching the sheep of a rich grazier and of subsequently setting fire to his house and barns.[38] He also quotes a very graphic illustration of planned, vengeful, and highly deliberate fire-raising in the case of Elizabeth Abbott. She announced that

> she had viewed the place where she resolved to do it, for she would get pitch and tar, and set fire in the mayor's shop, or in some other shop where there was lint and tow, and would stand by it that she might be taken and would own herself to have done it.[39]

There are one or two points of special interest in this case. The first concerns the deliberation with which the perpetrator went about her business; this was no spur of the moment event. The second concerns the manner in which she made no attempt to conceal her activities. One may speculate whether this was due to bravado, a feeling of imperviousness to control by the authorities, or to a degree of mild hypomania. We have no way of knowing and the motivation appears to be every bit as mixed as with a large number of contemporary cases. The motive of revenge may be directed towards a specific individual or individuals or it may be the expression of a more general vengeful feeling towards society. Such people may harbour vengeful feelings not unlike the monster in Mary Shelley's *Frankenstein* who said 'I am malicious because I am miserable'. It is a motive that also seems to cut across many of the other cases already described. It may be said to be the commonest of all motives, but this is not always apparent on first inspection of the case. Very careful and persistent exploration may be required before the motive emerges. In the survey of imprisoned arsonists referred to earlier, we found that motives of revenge predominated – in 38 cases out of a total of 113. In the media accounts of the case described in Vignette 17, it was suggested that the young man in question indulged in arson in order to get back at those he felt had been harassing him or who had received the advantages of a happy home life he felt had been denied him.

Fire-raising is not uncommon as a highly personal form of revenge against employers. Considerable damage may be caused to property by those who are seeking to redress some real or imagined wrong such as dismissal, or a reprimand, or the preferential treatment of others by management. Such employees may be very knowledgeable about the premises and how best to set the fire. Woodward quotes the case of a warehouseman who felt underpaid. He entered the warehouse late at night and set fire to the stock of basket wickerwork furniture. Ninety per cent of the premises and 20 per cent of an adjacent building were destroyed. During questioning he is said to have told the police that 'his original intention was only to cause trouble by changing labels on items which were to be shown at an exhibition; starting the fire was a last-minute decision.'[40] Reference has already been made in Chapter 3 to fires raised by school-children from vengeful motives. Occasionally, such offending appears to occur 'out of the blue', though *past* animosity towards teaching staff can sometimes be elicited. In these cases the arson is often associated with other demonstrations of aggression and anti-social conduct. Such phenomena are considered further in Chapter 6.

There is also a more generally vengeful group of adults which includes those who have a near-delusional mental state impervious to outside influence; their motives have much in common with the more psychotically motivated arsonists already described.

Vignette 18

A man aged about 30 had developed a passionate and quite unshakeable belief that a young woman was in love with him. His passions were not reciprocated; in fact they were actively resisted on several occasions. So obsessive were this man's amorous desires that they had some of the delusional qualities referred to earlier. As a means of gaining attention to his plight and of getting back at the young woman concerned he placed an incendiary device in her home with the avowed intention of killing her and her family. Fortunately, a family member spotted the device and dealt with it before the fire took too great a hold. Many years after this event, the offender (detained in hospital on a hospital order without time limit) still harboured vengeful feelings and seemed quite without insight into what he had done or compassion for his intended victims. It is important to stress here that the vengeful arsonist is likely to harbour his or her destructive desires over a long period.

Vignette 19

A woman tried to 'blow up her former lover's wife with a petrol bomb'. Having disguised herself as a man she placed the device under the victim's car. Earlier she had set another device with the aim of impaling her victim. The court heard that she had been receiving psychotherapy for her condition and that this needed to continue for a further period. She was made the subject of a probation order with a requirement that she continue her treatment and did not contact her former lover or his wife (*The Independent*, January 1, 1990, p. 3).

Vignette 20

A man in his late forties was sentenced to life imprisonment for killing his former girlfriend and her new lover by setting fire to their bed with petrol while they slept. The woman was burned beyond recognition and her lover died hours later in hospital from 100 per cent burns. The prosecution alleged that the defendant 'planned their killing out of revenge and jealousy'. He claimed that he was under the influence of anti-depressent medication at the time 'and was in a dream-like state'. The detective in charge of the case said 'what a terrible crime – and it could have been much worse. There were three other people in the house, so there could have been five bodies had it not been for the quick action by the fire service.' The case illustrates not only the seriousness of such offences but the manner in which they can affect persons other than the intended victims (*The Independent*, July 5, 1990, p. 4).

Vignette 21

A woman in her twenties started a fire in her bedroom intending to choke her lover to death. She told the court that she had started the fire in an attempt to get revenge for the repeated beatings she had received at his hands. She seemed to have placed the safety of her pet cat above that of her lover for she told the court that 'I decided to wake him . . . when I realised the cat might be trapped . . . I only wish I had left him in there . . . I only went back to get the cat.' She was placed on probation (*The Independent*, March 6, 1990, p. 3).

Sometimes acts of more general revenge involving arson occur when groups of people feel badly treated by the authorities. A recent press account describes how 'Hundreds of rioters set fire to buildings and cars in New York early today during . . . an outbreak of violence over the police killing of an Hispanic immigrant.' One thousand youths went on the rampage in which one person died, 25 were injured and cars, dwellings and shops burned (*Evening Standard*, July 8, 1992, p. 11). Such acts are grimly reminiscent of recent riots in parts of the UK.

It will be readily apparent from the case illustrations above that arson committed for reasons of revenge is a very worrying offence; the more so when we consider that of those arsonists who repeat their offences, a significant number are those whose motives were vengeful.[41]

Pyromania

I now consider a group of arsonists who do not appear to be suffering to a significant degree from any of the mental disorders described above or to be operating from clear motives of revenge. They seem to derive excitement and satisfaction from the involvement in fire-raising and in attending or busying themselves at the scene and calling out the fire brigade. Sometimes such persons are described as operating from a sense of 'heroics' or 'vanity'. These are the offenders who need to be at the centre of things and who demand attention. As indicated in Chapter 4, they may be spotted by an observant police or fire officer at more than one fire. It has been suggested that some volunteer firemen may have such fire-raising tendencies.

The history of the use of the term pyromania has been usefully described by Geller et al.[42] In the nineteenth century it was regarded as a form of monomania or insanity but later workers tended to dismiss this notion. The famous Henry Maudsley went as far as to state that it was a concept devised to hide 'inadequate observation under a pretentious name'.[43] In the 1920s interest in pyromania as a clinical entity was revived, largely as a result of the work of Freudian and Jungian psychoanalysts. One such analyst, Stekel, suggested there was a heavy sexual component to the condition.[44] The debate as to the usefulness of the term has swung backwards and forwards in recent years. Geller et al. suggest that the interest in pyromania is but an aspect of law and psychiatry's (often conflicting) interests in assigning responsibility for criminal behaviour, or rather gaining exculpation from it. In their words 'pyromania becomes a barometer of psychiatry's struggle with the individual's responsibility for his actions.'[45]

Pyromania is currently classified as a mental disorder in one of the standard works on classification, *The Diagnostic and Statistical Manual of Mental Disorders* (DSM, III Revised). It is described as follows:

> The essential features of this disorder are deliberate and purposeful (rather than accidental) fire-setting on more than one occasion; tension or affective arousal prior to setting the fires; and intense pleasure, gratification, a relief when setting the fires, with interest in, curiosity about, or attraction to fire and its situational context or associated

characteristics . . . the fire-setting is not done for monetary gain, as an expression of socio-political ideology, to conceal criminal activity, to express anger or vengeance, to improve one's living circumstances, or in response to a delusion or hallucination.[46]

The text also indicates that the behaviour is often pre-meditated; repetitive; the individual may watch fires, may leave clues, raise false alarms and be indifferent to the consequences of the fire for life and property; he or she may obtain satisfaction from the resulting destruction.[47]

Lewis and Yarnell, in a somewhat shorter statement, identified pyromaniacs as a group of individuals who repeatedly raise fires for no practical reason other than an irresistible impulse to do so, and 'perhaps some sort of sensual satisfaction obtained from the fire and associated events'.[48] In a recent and interesting paper which examines pyromania from a clinical perspective, Geller suggests that a better description for some persistent arsonists would be that of 'communicative arson'.[49] He means by this that pathological fire-raising can be seen as a means of communicating a wish, a desire or a need. Such a view would be much in accord with Winnicott's view of the 'antisocial tendency'. Winnicott says that 'The antisocial tendency is characterized by an *element in it which compels the environment to be important* [italics in original]. The patient through unconscious drives compels someone to attend to management.'[50] Such an assumption is a useful working concept for those who have to deal with persistent arsonists.

A fairly classic case of pyromania is described below.

Vignette 22

A woman in her late forties was initially praised as a heroine for her apparent efforts to rescue two children from a house fire. Later, she was to admit that she had started the blaze herself; she was jailed for life, having pleaded guilty to manslaughter and five counts of arson. Her history, as given in court, revealed that she had started fires on three previous occasions. She was described by the prosecuting counsel as someone who had a compulsive fascination for lighting fires, obtaining excitement by watching the arrival of the fire brigade. She also plagued the authorities with hoax phone calls. She was described as not being very bright and by her counsel as 'suffering from an illness, a sickness . . . in respect of which there appears to be no medical treatment . . . she is not evil in the normally accepted sense.' Commenting on the case and others, Dr Angus Campbell, a respected forensic psychiatrist, suggested that many pyromaniacs suffered from serious personality disorder. 'This sort of behaviour often originates in one fire which gives the person a buzz and gets them hooked.' He describes how he once treated an auxiliary fireman 'who always dashed to the seat of the flames, naturally reaping accolades. Eventually, after fighting seven or eight fires, it was discovered that he was starting them himself' (*The Independent*, June 12, 1992, pp. 1 and 2).

Vignette 23

A man with a long previous history of fire-raising was charged with setting fire to a friend's house. He also had a history of making many hoax telephone calls to both the police and the fire services. He received a health care disposal – being made subject to a hospital order with restrictions without time limit under the Mental Health Act. Originally thought to be of limited intelligence, he was found to be brighter and responsive to moderately intensive psychotherapy. During this it emerged that from an early age he had become excited by the sight of firemen in uniform. He was eventually transferred from a secure hospital to a local psychiatric facility and seemed to be doing quite well.

Sexually motivated arson

Ever since Freud and his followers drew upon ancient myth to sugest a link between the sexual act and arson there have been numerous accounts in the psychoanalytic literature which have tended to support this view. However, such accounts are largely anecdotal and have tended to be repeated in learned journals over the years, thus giving a false credibility to a somewhat suspect concept. Some workers, for example Rice and Harris, have been heavily critical of psychoanalytic theorising;[51] and Foust, somewhat more positively, has stressed the need for careful clinical evaluation of individual cases.[52] One of the most sensible perspectives on the topic is provided by Fras:

> Adult fire-setters [pyromaniacs] . . . represent a hetero-geneous group in terms of motivation and psychodynamics . . . they feel unbearable tension, which is released by setting the fire and watching it. Sexual excitement is sometimes described, but not necessarily so. Others derive need fulfillment through the process of extinguishing the flames, with its masculine symbolism. Both types of fire-setters may have histories of sexual humiliation and general feelings of inferiority, with fire restoring power and a kind of strong symbolic fulfillment, either by the act of setting the fire or extinguishing it since both activities have enormous social effects as well.[53]

Fras makes the point that such behaviour has strong similarities to sex offending. 'In its compulsive, stereotyped sequence of mounting pressure, pyromania resembles the sexual perversions, as it may parallel them in its imperviousness to treatment.'[54] The important place given by Fras to sexual problems finds some confirmation in Hurley and Manahan's study of imprisoned arsonists. They found that 54 per cent of the men had clear psychosexual difficulties and marital problems and 60 per cent reported difficulties in social relationships with women.[55] In his classic psychoanalytic account of a case of 'incendiarism', Simmel describes a young man, George, aged 21, who was referred to him for his compulsive fire-raising behaviour.[56] During analysis Simmel discovered that this young man had not had any kind of sexual experience other than a temporary period of masturbation at the age of 8 or 9. His background was disturbed and his parents were divorced; he was reared by very strict and somewhat cruel grandparents. Having caught him masturbating they threatened to cut off his penis. Despite this he continued to do so, but amidst great feelings of guilt and anxiety. Soon after this he was hospitalised for peritonitis and as part of his post-operative treatment was given an enema by his grandmother. Following a re-awakening of sexual impulses in adolescence his grandparents forbade him to associate with girls until he was 25, considering all forms of pre-marital intercourse sinful. Eventually, his father re-married and George went to live with him and his stepmother. He related well to her, and she gave him advice on sexual and related matters. However, Simmel concludes that this well-meaning advice and help was probably seductive in nature and re-awakened repressed infantile masturbatory impulses. He dealt with the tension produced by these by indulging in repetitive acts of setting fire to plots of grass. Simmel also suggests that George unconsciously *wanted* to be caught,

> for in all his acts of incendiarism he also used his father's automobile to drive to the vacant lots. This car was painted red and was very conspicuous. He drove the car onto the lot, set fire to the dry grass, then drove away from the lot, called the fire department and waited near the fire for the firemen. Naturally not only he personally, but his car as well became conspicuous.[57]

Simmel's account of aetiology is expressed in classic psycho-analytic terms:

> In conclusion we can say that George repressed his impulses toward genital masturbation out of his fear of the threatened castration. He sought an inner escape from this conflict by regressing to the urethral phase of his libidinal development. Whenever his bladder was full, he produced an erection, which was relieved by urinating. Now, in a symbolic repetition of this process, George felt the compulsive need to splash water on the fire, thus to extinguish an excitation which he himself had kindled.[58]

I am not advocating uncritical espousal of this classic psycho-analytic exploration and explanation; my purpose has merely been to show that in a number of cases the compulsion to raise fires *may* have very complex and deep-seated roots. These are only likely to be available for resolution if a productive relationship is established over a lengthy period of time with whomever is assigned to deal with the individual. The case also illustrates the not uncommon feature of compulsive arsonists' tendency to place themselves in a situation where they may be caught out in their activities.

Vignette 24

This concerned a man in his mid-forties, detained in a secure hospital. He suffered from both a degree of mental impairment and from psychopathic (personality) disorder. He had a long history of arson offences, some of them quite serious. He had always claimed to have obtained sexual arousal and occasional orgasm from watching the fires he set. But perhaps of more significance was his additional predilection for the mutilation of the cadavers of both sexes. His case was indicative of gross psychopathology and illustrates the overlap between different categories of anti-social conduct – in this case, the molestation of corpses.

Young adult vandalism and fire-raising

The backgrounds and motivations of adolescent and young adult fire-raisers appear to be rather different from those characterising children who raise fires. They form a separate group and are considered in Chapter 6. The adolescents and younger adults we looked at in our prison sample seemed to have been motivated more specifically by boredom and to have engaged in the behaviour for 'kicks'. It is not unknown for bored young employees to set fire to their places of work. Cases have been reported in the hotel and catering industry.[59] In some cases, there was also an accompanying element of getting back at a society that did not appear to care about them. Unlike child fire-raisers, the backgrounds of young adult arsonists seemed less socially and psychologically disturbed. It is also important to note that the arson offences committed by this age group are often closely associated with the ingestion of alcohol. The following case example shows how some of these elements may be combined.

Vignette 25

A group of five unemployed older teenagers (ages ranging from 16 to 19) had been to a disco where they had imbibed a fair amount of alcohol, though they were not drunk. They had waited for a considerable time for the last bus home only to find they had missed it. They had been whiling away their time at the bus stop indulging in a fair amount of horse-play. As they became more impatient, their horse-play escalated into more aggressive activity. They smashed the windows of a large outfitter's shop nearby, entered it, and began damaging the contents. In the course of this activity, one of them lit some waste paper while others looked on encouraging him. A fire soon took hold engulfing the premises and rapidly destroying the shop and its contents.

MANAGEMENT

'Their candles are all out'
Macbeth, Act II, Scene i

It will be obvious from the range of explanations and motives outlined in this chapter that no single form of management will be effective. But because fire-raising behaviour is so diverse, and because, as already suggested, motives may be obscure, it is very important that each case receives full analysis; this is particularly important when we come to consider the risk of re-offending, which I shall discuss shortly. The classification I have outlined, for all its acknowledged deficiencies, should be of some help in enabling us to distinguish between those arsonists who engage in their offence for purely fraudulent motives, those who are politically motivated and those whose behaviour is vandalistic; those whose behaviour is motivated by clear evidence of mental disorder of one kind or another and those whose motivation is more difficult to get to grips with, the vengeful and the so-called pyromaniacs.

Predominantly non-mentally disordered arsonists

In these cases a full investigation of the social and personal circumstances of the individual concerned is valuable in order to rule out any significant psycho-pathological factors. As already indicated, an arsonist motivated by apparently fraudulent motives may be suffering from a degree of depression and this may be responsive to remedial measures even if a prison sentence is imposed. The same considerations apply to some politically motivated arsonists; it would be a mistake to rule out the possibility that within their ranks there are a small number who are suffering from a degree of mental disturbance, although not perhaps of a degree to fulfil a formal clinical psychiatric diagnosis. Apart from these considerations, politically motivated arsonists and those driven by a general urge to be destructive (the vandals) are best dealt with through general penal and other measures available. However, the wider implications of their behaviour are matters for more general consideration by politicians and by governments, and it would be inappropriate to offer opinion on these matters in a book of this kind. Nevertheless, it *is* important to set such behaviours in the broader social context of violence in society more generally. Anthony Storr has some apposite comments in this respect:

> it is clear that violent crime will persist to some degree in any large society, since we cannot cure, eliminate, or prevent the birth of all individuals deemed to be suffering from aggressive personality disorder. However the evidence does suggest that by far the majority of violent offences are committed by people from the lower levels of society, in which individuals are most likely to feel neglected, unappreciated, and of no account. Any measures which reduce inequality, alleviate poverty, and provide socially valued work, and which therefore raise self-esteem, are likely to reduce the level of violence.[60]

Mentally disordered fire-raisers

Those arsonists who engage in their activities because of serious psychiatric disturbance may well respond to treatment for their underlying illness. Medication, if taken regularly, may help to keep their most acute and intrusive hallucinations or delusions at bay. Faulk says: 'in the case of the patient whose perception has been distorted by mental illness, one can treat this and reasonably expect him to stay safe, certainly as long as the illness does not return.'[61] One of the problems that arises is the degree to which compliance with medication is continued by the patient once discharged to the community. The cases described by Carpenter and King and by Byrne and Walsh show that medication for an organic condition such as epilepsy or some form of hormonal imbalance may also be most helpful; indeed, as the cases show, it may change not only the outcome but also the diagnosis. Medication may also be helpful for some mentally impaired arsonists whose behaviour is aggressively impulsive. It is here that effective social and psychiatric supervision is essential. For those whose offences have merited a hospital order with restrictions, a period of parole or life licence, then such supervision is mandatory and provides supervisors with sanctions. For those who are discharged without such sanctions, supervision is not likely to be as effective; such persons have a low rating at present within the structures of community mental health after-care. However, one is hopeful that the various reports produced by sub-groups working under the chairman-ship of Dr John Reed of the Department of Health will not only raise consciousness of mental health after-care needs of offender-patients more generally, but also have an impact upon the need to provide 'ring-fenced' funding for a group of people who are often 'unloved, unloving and unlovely'.[62] One of the most critical problems is that of accommodation (and this applies to all convicted of what we might perhaps describe as 'pathological arson'). Hostels are understandably very reluctant to take known fire-raisers, not only for reasons of safety and the protection of other residents, but because insurance cover may be difficult to obtain or maintain. It is sad, but perhaps understandable, that some workers will endeavour to hide the fact that a client or patient has a history of arson (if their most recent offence is for something else) in order to gain a residential place. Serious thought needs to be given to the provision of special facilities enhanced by regular and intensive psychiatric and psychological support. At present such provision is extremely rare.

It would be a mistake to believe that formal psychotherapy of varying degrees of intensity has no place in the management of psychotic or psychopathic arsonists detained in hospital. Cox has carried out much interesting long-term group work with psychotic offender-patients (including arsonists) detained in Broadmoor Hospital. Such work requires considerable skills and imagination if one is to become tuned in to what such offender-patients are trying to communicate. Cox says:

> An arsonist may be able to relive his experience of setting fire to the house of his ex-'flame', who had jilted him, in the presence of therapist A (a non-arsonist); whereas therapist B (also a non-arsonist) 'would not understand'.

He asks:

> What does this mean? It implies that there must be empathic understanding between therapist A, which is not present with therapist B. There will be other occasions when therapist B will be able to receive what the patient says, whereas therapist A will not.[63]

Elsewhere Cox demonstrates the helpful elements that are present within a group psychotherapeutic setting:

This means that a disclosure from one patient is frequently followed almost immediately by similar disclosures from other patients, 'I was waiting for you to start so that I could join in' . . . 'Funny, I was just going to say that.' In actual fact, the patient who was '*just* going to say that' was a reticent arsonist, terrified of making personal disclosures. But when, after eighteen months in another group, another patient admitted that he was an arsonist, the certainty of not being the odd man out allowed him to say something that he had 'just' been going to say![64]

Describing another case, Cox suggests that

His arson was no substitute sexual activity, but rather a way of getting his family, highly respectable and respected in the local Cornish village, into the headlines of the local paper, by ensuring that the reporters knew of his activity: 'Fancy one of them doing that. They were always such a good family.'[65]

One of the advantages of such an approach with a range of offender-patients suffering from varied psychiatric conditions is that it reinforces the importance of carefully examining the *individual* case. Elsewhere Cox says:

The arsonist may be diagnosed as subnormal, neurotic, psychotic, or psychopathic. The act may be of profound symbolic importance to the patient or almost incidental. It may be of overt sexual significance, and the patient will claim that he had his best orgasm as he watched the flames leaping up, or that his greatest moment of sexual excitement was when he was helping the fire service unsuccessfully to put out the fire which he had started . . . . On other occasions the act may be symbolically associated with love or hate. ('My best flame, you set me on fire, burning anger . . . '). The arsonist may show psychotic concrete thinking so that self-immolation occurred when Charles Wesley's hymn, 'Kindle a flame of sacred love on the mean altar of my heart' was taken literally.[66]

Cox goes on to stress a point made earlier that 'the almost

limitless range of clinical presentations means there is no neat unitary hypothesis which can underlie the behaviour of all patients convicted of arson.'[67]

Vengeful and other fire-raisers

As will readily be seen, the sub-classifications made here are somewhat artificial and I would ask readers to bear in mind Cox's injunction above. If we accept the fact that a number of vengeful arsonists and pyromaniacs may commit their offences because they feel wronged or misunderstood, any attempts to help them to explore such alleged wrongs may be useful. Attempts can then be made to find ways in which they may achieve more satisfaction from their life's experiences. Since we know that many of them are socially inept, and that they set fires in order to draw attention to themselves, techniques aimed at improving their self-regard, self-image and social competence should help to minimise the risk of future offending. This might best be achieved by specific social skills training such as the development of legitimate forms of social assertiveness, since we know from the work of Jackson *et al.* and others that a number of arsonists have problems in asserting themselves in an acceptable manner.[68] Jackson *et al.* suggest that 'factors which militate against alternative behaviours to arson may be equally as important to a thorough analysis of [the fire-raiser's] pathological behaviour, as those factors which directly promote the use of fire.'[69] The serious 'assertion deficits' in arsonists have also been noted by Harris and Rice.[70]

The need for a multi-disciplinary and multi-causal approach is demonstrated very ably in a recent paper by Clare *et al.*[71] The authors adopted a cognitive-behavioural approach to the management of a 23-year-old man suffering from psychopathic disorder. He had been previously convicted of two charges of arson and spent four and a half years in a special hospital. At the time of the study he was resident in a specialist psychiatric facility catering for patients with learning disabilities and severe behavioural problems. Most patients in the unit stayed for about eighteen months. This patient was subjected to a very careful multi-disciplinary assessment. Sadly, he had been born with a harelip and a cleft palate. These had been badly repaired leaving him speech impaired. In addition, he suffered from a mild degree of mental impairment (learning disability). He was unhappy about his appearance but in the past had declined offers of surgery. In his early teens he had begun to make hoax telephone calls to the fire service and followed this by two acts of arson. On the first occasion he had been placed under a supervision order and on the second he was made the subject of a hospital order with restrictions under the Mental Health Act. His therapists formulated a multi-faceted approach that would aim to enhance his social skills, improve his educational standard and offer a programme of desensitisation to impulses to engage in fire-raising conduct. (This was carried out by graded exposure over several months to holding matches.) He also agreed to undergo facial surgery and to accept plans for later operations to improve his speech. However, he was still considered to be vulnerable to engagement in fire-raising behaviour. Because of this, controlled situations were devised in which he was subjected to the arousal of negative feelings and stress. Over a long period of time he was taught coping mechanisms to deal with these. Eventually he was able to use these independently of his therapist's interventions. These were said to be especially useful in situations in which he felt put down or unwanted. He was able subsequently to undertake a part-time job (despite some lapses in attendance) and to form a relationship with a member of the opposite sex. During his stay in the facility no instances of hoax calls or fire-raising behaviour were said to have occurred despite some acknow-ledged temptation to do so on the patient's part. At the time of last follow-up (some four years later) he was in full-time work, had formed an apparently mutually happy relationship with his girl-friend, had been conditionally discharged from his restriction order and was living in the open community. No further instances of fire-raising behaviour had been reported, though on two occasions, when under stress, he had felt tempted to engage in such behaviour. The authors concluded that 'his recent success in forming an intimate relationship and in gaining paid employment, both of which will alleviate his social isolation, provide some cause for optimism that he will not engage in fire setting again'.[72]

Several important points emerge from this seminal piece of work. First, the importance of careful assessment, if necessary, over a prolonged period. Second, the need to adopt a multi-causal approach to the problem presented by such offenders. This is likely to involve the willing collaboration of a range of professionals from a variety of disciplines. Third, such management is a time-consuming business; it requires patience and tenacity. Fourth, because of this, it is labour intensive and costly. However, such expense needs to be set against the costs for all concerned in both human and economic terms of further instances of fire-raising.

THE ASSESSMENT OF RISK

Although only a small proportion of male arsonists sentenced to short-term prison sentences are reconvicted of arson over a short time-span, men sentenced to longer terms have a much higher rate of reconviction. Workers in special hospitals also describe similar reconviction rates for hospitalised arsonists. Faulk has suggested, on the basis of a number of studies in the literature, that as far as prisoners are concerned, 50 per cent of those sentenced to a long period of imprisonment for arson are likely to commit another destructive offence, not merely arson. He goes on to state that

> Although I have suggested that it may not be possible to tell whether a particular person will commit arson again, and furthermore, the chances overall of a repeat are low, one is obliged to estimate the chances of him once more doing something destructive. Most importantly, one must estimate in what *situation* and under what *conditions* this might be [italics added].[73]

I have written extensively elsewhere on the assessment of dangerousness in offenders and offender-patients.[74] Suffice it to say that, as with other serious offenders, arsonists require to be looked at under a number of headings: their past behaviours, both criminal and otherwise; full details of previous and index offences; trigger factors; presence or otherwise of mental disorder; the degree to which the arsonist is still in a situation of vulnerability; self-perceptions; capacity to cope with provocation; acknowledgement of the facts of what they have done; and a capacity for forming some kind of relationship with a 'therapist'. Dr Peter Scott wrote what is probably the seminal paper on this topic.[75] Perhaps the last word on basic assessment should rest with him.

It is patience, thoroughness and persistence in this process [of data collection], rather than any diagnostic or interviewing brilliance that produces results. In this sense, the telephone, the written request for past records and the checking of information against other informants, are the important diagnostic devices. Having collected the facts under the headings of (1) the offence; (2) past behaviour; (3) personal data; (4) social circumstances, it is useful to scan them from a number of different directions with a view to answering certain key questions relating to dangerousness.[76]

CONCLUSION

In this chapter I have sought to outline a classification of adult fire-raisers but acknowledge that such classifications are imperfect in many ways. It is hoped that the behaviours and attitudes demonstrated by the fire-raisers I have described have been brought alive by the case vignettes provided. Management must be based not only upon a detailed and empathic understanding of each case, but also upon the possibilities inherent in a multi-disciplinary approach in which dogmatic ideologies have no place. Arson is a particularly dangerous crime; for the following reasons. First, as I have shown in previous chapters, it is not easily detected and many cases probably go undetected. Second, it is an offence that can be committed with comparative ease, and at one remove from the victim. Third, even if a single victim is intended for attack, there is always the strong possibility that others may be injured or killed in the ensuing conflagration. Fourth, motivation is often obscure and it is all too easy to be misled by superficial explanations for the crime. Fifth, although the assessment of risk of repetition is extremely difficult, careful attention to a detailed assessment of facts and attitudes may make it less so. Finally, within the present state of the art, those who are concerned in making decisions about future behaviour can only try to make a judgement based upon a detailed and careful evaluation of the *individual case*.

6

CHILD FIRE-RAISERS: MOTIVES AND MANAGEMENT

'Train up a child in the way he should go: and when he is old,
he will not depart from it.'

Proverbs, 22: 6

'And thus the child imposes on the Man'
Dryden, 'The Hind and the Panther', III: 389

INTRODUCTION

Readers may wonder why a separate chapter is being devoted to
fire-raising by children since, although there are probably as
many differences in the causes and manifestation of fire-raising
in children as there are in adults, they have much in common.
There are three reasons for doing so. First, a number of adult
arsonists have begun their fire-raising careers as children; thus
the seeds of such behaviour are sown early in life and we need
more detailed information about this. Second, the phenomenon
of fire-raising in childhood sometimes illustrates very clearly
the psychodynamic aspects of the behaviour. Third, early
intervention may provide a useful form of prophylaxis, and this
aspect leads us usefully into my final area of discussion in this
book – preventive measures. In England and Wales children
under 10 are not held to be criminally responsible for their acts so
that it is not strictly correct to write of arson in young children;
fire-raising is the preferred term. Other jurisdictions throughout
the world have similar provisions for excluding young children
from criminal proceedings, though almost everywhere children
who commit criminal acts may be subject to proceedings for their
own protection and/or the protection of others.

BRIEF REVIEW OF THE LITERATURE

There have been a number of surveys of fire-raising behaviour in children, perhaps the most famous being those published by Yarnell in 1940 and Lewis and Yarnell in 1951.[1] Unfortunately these two seminal works lacked control groups of normal children. As we shall see, nearly all the studies point to a high degree of psycho-social pathology in the backgrounds of these young deviants, and they seem to show a number of characteristics not demonstrated in non-delinquent children and in a number of delinquents not involved in arson.

One of the most interesting and fairly large-scale studies of fire-raising in a 'normal' population was that carried out by Ditsa Kafry in Berkeley, California, in the late 1970s.[2] She investigated the fire behaviour and knowledge in a random sample of ninety-nine boys of approximately 8 years of age. Children and parents were interviewed in their own homes and the latter were asked to complete a research questionnaire. The interviews and the questionnaires provided demographic data, child-rearing practices and information about fire behaviour. Kafry found that interest in fire was almost universal and 'fire-play' was carried out by 45 per cent of the boys studied. Kafry's findings tend to confirm the earlier views of Lewis and Yarnell that the 'incidence of children who play with fire is far greater than any statistics show'.[3] She also found that interest in fire began at a very early age – 18 per cent of fires set in Kafry's sample were raised before the age of 3. An equally ominous finding was that although the children's parents seemed aware of the risks of fires, a large percentage did not provide any adequate instruction and warning to their children. In Kafry's survey those children who played with matches and raised fires seemed to be more mischievous, aggressive, exhibitionistic and impulsive than those who expressed no such interest; such findings again confirm the earlier work of researchers such as Lewis and Yarnell. They are also of interest because they seem to be the same characteristics that are demonstrated in a number of adult arsonists, particularly those of aggression and impulsiveness. As far as family backgrounds were concerned, Kafry found that the homes of those boys who experimented with fire tended to be characterised by a greater degree of emotional and social deprivation; fathers played a less important role (or were absent) and mothers were frequently left to cope with the child-rearing. The fathers were often perceived to have a negative relationship with their sons (a finding commonly found in the backgrounds of children involved in other kinds of delinquency).

Some confirmation of Kafry's findings may be found in a study carried out by Stewart and Culver.[4] They examined forty-six children who had each raised at least one fire and had been admitted to a psychiatric ward, so they were not a 'normal' sample. The children were followed up after one to five years. Seven of the children, all boys, who were less than 13 years of age, were still raising fires, but they were held to be less serious than the ones they had raised before treatment. The authors considered that the persistent fire-raisers seemed to come from the less stable homes and to be more generally anti-social on follow-up than the children who no longer raised fires. However, they are the first to admit that their study did not enable them to predict with any degree of certainty which children would continue to raise fires.

Jacobson reached somewhat similar conclusions.[5] He examined the backgrounds and symptomatology of 104 child fire-raisers referred to an inner London child psychiatric clinic between 1973 and 1981. He compared the cases with a matched control group of non-fire-raisers. He considered that fire-raisers formed a sub-group of severe conduct disorders; they were younger than other character disordered children – and the peak age for their behaviour was 8. Their backgrounds seemed to be characterised by parental criminality, poor supervision and harsh or incon-sistent discipline with considerable family discord or disruption. Males predominated in the order of 5:1. He found that the often repeated assertion that there is an association between fire-raising, sexual disturbance and enuresis was not evident in his sample.

Unlike adult fire-raisers, fire-raising in childhood is not often associated with formal mental illness. However, there are some rare instances reported in the literature. Everall and LeCouteur describe briefly a case of fire-raising in a boy suffering from Asperger's syndrome – a rare developmental disorder akin to childhood autism. In this case, the boy had started his interest in fire-raising at an early age. Several of his episodes of fire-raising were apparently carefully planned. His home-life was charac-terised by caring parents, but his father was often away for long periods due to the nature of his employment; his mother was mainly responsible for his upbringing. Sadly, his expressions of remorse for his conduct did not entirely convince the professionals charged with caring for him. In addition, he appeared indifferent to the effects of his actions upon others. Such behaviour did not augur well for his capacity to desist from future fire-raising behaviour.[6]

As with adult fire-raisers, those workers with a psychoanalytic orientation have also concerned themselves with fire-raising in children. In an early paper Macht and Mack suggest that careful consideration should be given to the severe psychopathology that exists in many of these cases. They take the view that, in the first place,

> the act of setting a fire is a highly complex and determined piece of behaviour and not simply the product of the breakthrough of an impulse. It reflects . . . the expression of instinctual elements of destructiveness and libidinal excitement. Second . . . the fire-setting behaviour proved to have multiple determinants for the fire-setter in terms of the meaning of the act and its specific association with important human relationships both in the past and in the present. Third, the fire-setters regarded their act with *some* guilt and anxiety but did not consider the behaviour as entirely alien to them [italics added].

In their view 'fire-setting appears in this respect to have an intermediate status between a neurotic symptom and more conventional psychopathic behaviour.'[7]

Vandersall and Weiner studied twenty children who raised fires. Their findings were very similar to those of Macht and Mack. They were unable to find any consistent precipitating stresses, leading them to conclude that the fire-raising behaviour arose very much out of the child's inner conflicts. They discerned a sense of exclusion and loneliness amongst their subjects and unfulfilled dependency needs. This is, again, an interesting finding, since such features are not uncommon in some of the adult arsonists described in the previous chapter.[8]

Prediction

Vandersall and Weiner suggest that prediction requires a careful examination of the total inner and outer needs of the child.

Stewart and Culver, in the paper already referred to, state that 'the conclusion we draw is that the short-term prognosis of fire-raising in young children, at least in those who are admitted to a child psychiatry ward, is only fair and that there are no reliable ways as yet to tell whether a child will stop setting fires or continue.'[9] Heath *et al.* conclude somewhat ruefully:

> It is noteworthy that there are unfortunately no follow-up studies of childhood fire-setters. This omission certainly contributes to our continuing lack of knowledge in regard to the predictive value of this behaviour in childhood for adult adjustment.[10]

They also suggest that

> a comprehensive epidemiological study of childhood fire-setters which would provide data regarding incidence and prevalence, as well as clarify the relationship between childhood fire-setting and such demographic variables as sex, age, socio-economic status, race and family size is definitely needed.[11]

TOWARDS A CLASSIFICATION AND PRESCRIPTION FOR MANAGEMENT

In 1984, two American researchers, Wooden and Berkey, published what is probably one of the most comprehensive studies of young fire-raisers to have appeared since the early work of Lewis and Yarnell.[12] Moreover, they used a control group of 'normal' subjects. This study is now described in a little detail; where I consider it helpful, I have interspersed *their* data with vignettes drawn from a variety of other sources.

The investigators tried to distinguish the *behavioural characteristics* of juvenile fire-raisers, the several *types* of fire-raisers and their *motives* (cf. Chapter 5). The study consists of a survey of sixty-nine juvenile fire-raisers apprehended during a four-year period – 1979 to 1983 – in Southern California. They were compared with a group of seventy-eight non-fire-raisers. Plans to have a third same-size group of delinquents not convicted of arson had to be abandoned because of technical difficulties. They also examined the work of 128 fire-fighters involved in a programme for rehabilitating juvenile fire-raisers. This would

79

appear to be the first occasion on which fire-fighters have been questioned as to their own backgrounds and motives.

General characteristics of the children

As with other researchers, Wooden and Berkey found among the fire-raising children poor family relationships; warring parents; a significant degree of sexual abuse, particularly, but by no means exclusively, among their female juvenile fire-raisers (a feature not noted significantly in previous studies; maybe because before our current interest in the problem the question was never explored); poor peer relationships; poor assertive skills; and multiple behavioural problems. They make the very interesting and insightful comment that 'these youngsters wait until they are literally "burned out", and then they light something.'[13] One of the key features that distinguished the group of juvenile fire-raisers from other delinquents in Wooden and Berkey's study was that the former group consisted predominantly of *middle-class Caucasian* males. In the latter group, poor black youngsters featured significantly. Helpfully, they distinguish three age groups – *younger children*, 4–8; *pre-teenagers*, 9–12; *teenagers*, 13–17. They identify four useful categories of fire-raising youngsters:

1 Curiosity leading to fire – the 'playing with matches fire-setter' identified by Kafry.[14] Such youngsters were not bent on destruction. They seemed to come from homes where supervision and control in relation to the use of fire were somewhat lacking.

Vignette 1

An example illustrating this form of behaviour is drawn not from Wooden and Berkey but, somewhat surprisingly, from a frank statement about his early interest in fire-raising by a well-known English actor, Michael York. In an article in *The Independent* of November 4, 1991 (p.16), he describes his early childhood fascination and curiosity about fire.

> I took advantage of being brought up in a mostly matriarchal society because my father was away in the war, and I was this tiny tyrant, adventurous and naughty at the same time. . . . I loved bonfires . . . I became fascinated by

fire . . . I loved the incandescent beauty. . . . I was an absolute arsonist – a little kind of Nazi – I burnt my father's library: my mother came down once, horrified to see me in the act of book burning, and literally the whole fireplace was filled with books, smouldering and blazing away.

He describes how 'fire still haunts me'. 'I remember in New York seeing a liquor store go up, which stopped me in my tracks. I was absolutely spell-bound.'[15] Michael York's very frank account of his behaviour as a child reveals not only the curiosity about fire indicated by a number of workers, but its potential dangers. It is also illustrative of the continuation of the fascination referred to in Chapter 2.

2 Young fire-raisers who are motivated by anger at adverse home environments and harbour feelings of rejection and/or neglect – the 'cry for help' fire-raisers.

Vignette 2

Wooden and Berkey describe the case of 'Jerry', aged 8. He had lost his mother a year before his fire-raising incident and his father had been re-married for six months. The weekend before he set his fire his grandfather had died. Jerry had recently become withdrawn, disobedient and was not doing well in junior school. He is said to have day-dreamed about fire by day and dreamed about his dead mother at night. The fire he raised involved the ignition of his father's second wedding pictures. To the authors this seemed a clear case of a 'cry for help'.

Vignette 3

In another case, Wooden and Berkey record how a boy of 3 years of age set fire to the cribs in which his 1-year-old twin sisters were resting. 'The boy apparently took a calendar off the wall, put it on the lighted gas stove and threw it into the babies' cribs.'[16]

3 Older youngsters who engaged in arson as a pattern of juvenile delinquency. These were youngsters who responded to peer-group pressures, claimed excitement from their escapades, indulged in other acts of vandalism and did not foresee the consequences of their acts.

Vignette 4

With others, a boy of 14 set fire to his school. He dropped a lighted match into a bottle of turpentine. The school went up in flames very speedily causing damage worth £80,000. His conduct was seen to be connected with a wider range of behaviour disturbances. He was placed under supervision and required to attend an educational course run by the local social services department and the fire service. This course is the subject of later comment (*The Independent*, July 14, 1992, p. 13).

4   The pathological juvenile fire-raiser who sets fires repetitively, frequently and in a ritualistic fashion – the near-equivalent of the adult pyromaniac.

It is interesting to note that the parental attitudes in these cases also seem sometimes to be quite pathological. The history of one such fire-raiser in Wooden and Berkey's sample revealed that as a small child his mother had been amused by and encouraged him in his attempt to light cigarettes.

Vignette 5

This is a short account of the career of a young man who attained great publicity as a juvenile fire-raiser and subsequently as an adult arsonist. He is said to have set his first fire, to a toy aeroplane, at the age of 3. He is also said to have tried to set fires in the family home. At the age of 10 he again set fire to the house; he is said to have claimed that he thought the house was empty, but in fact his father was indoors and had to be rescued from the roof. Some time later, he returned to the house – by then a gutted wreck, and tried to set fire to it again. At the age of 8 he had tried to set fire to a church having been reproved by the nuns for 'not praying'. He is said to have stated that 'I just liked the flames.' He was sent to various residential establishments and was again in trouble when he absconded on more than one occasion. At the age of 15 he was sent to a secure psychiatric hospital. Following transfer to less secure conditions he was eventually discharged into the community. Hindsight seems to indicate that he was not as ready for the outside world as had been hoped. From early childhood the media had expressed an interest in his case and had made a film about him. Subsequently, a further film was made about his career as an adult. It has been suggested that this diet of media interest was a bit too rich for him and that he suffered as a result. His relationship with a woman who had befriended him went through a number of bad patches; he drank heavily and suffered bouts of depression. During one of these bad periods he set fire to a bottling plant, causing damage amounting to several hundred thousand pounds. At his trial, the psychiatric reports on him were said to have been negative, largely concentrating on his apparent untreatability, and he received a sentence of life imprisonment. At the time the article about him was published an appeal was being considered (*The Independent on Sunday*, August 4, 1991).[17]

MANAGEMENT

As with the adult arsonist, the juvenile fire-raiser will be more likely to respond to management if this is based upon a careful analysis of needs. This can only be achieved if all the social, familial and emotional factors are carefully assessed and an attempt made at some kind of classification, as described previously in somewhat rudimentary fashion. For the very young fire-raiser, a programme of education aimed at an understanding of the dangers of fire would seem most appropriate. Such education would also need to include the parents since a number of them appear to be quite oblivious to the need to teach children about the dangers of fire.

In less tractable cases an approach based upon behaviour modification techniques has apparently met with some degree of success. Holland has described the treatment of a 7-year-old boy, in which he was rewarded financially for not striking matches. The fire-raising behaviour is said to have been eliminated with no recurrence at an eight-month follow-up.[18] Welsh used a technique known as satiation on two 7-year-old boys. They spent their therapeutic sessions – lasting over an hour and a half on each occasion – lighting matches under controlled conditions. It is important to point out that this approach also had a highly aversive component. In one case, the child was required to hold the match until the heat could be felt on the finger-tips; in the other, the child was required to hold the match at arm's length until fatigue intervened.[19] Follow-up revealed that there was no recurrence at six months. In both these examples, follow-up was short and some may think that the methods used were somewhat draconian. The provision of facilities for young fire-raisers to light fires under carefully controlled conditions has been described by Wooden and Berkey in their study and by workers at Aycliffe – a centre for highly disturbed children in the north of England. 'During one session a young arsonist may be asked to start and then tackle a real but controlled blaze – in a frying pan for example – with . . . cakes as a reward for prompt action' (*The Independent on Sunday*, August 4, 1991).

In Vignette 4, reference was made to a special course run by a social services department and the local fire service. On this course, young fire-raisers are vigorously confronted with the effects of their behaviour. The experience is very intensive and the young people find it very demanding. In some cases they are required to write letters of apology to those persons or those whose property has been the object of their attacks. In addition to these activities, they view videos on the effects of fire, they meet fire-fighters and engage in a variety of board games (graded according to age) aimed at bringing the dangers of fire home to them. Other youngsters, at centres such as Aycliffe, receive intensive counselling on a group and an individual basis. Some of them require a great deal of help in expressing their hostility and in developing adequate social skills that enable them to deal with life's stresses in less inflammatory ways. Working with the family as a group has proved to be successful in some cases. In his book on family therapy, the distinguished family therapist Salvador Minuchin describes work undertaken by one of his colleagues with a family in which the 'fire-setter' appeared to be the 'scape-goat' for the rest of the family's complex problems. Minuchin conveys skilfully the need to carefully explore the problems and perspectives of the family as a whole.[20]

Techniques similar to those used in the UK are in use in the United States; a number of these are described in Wooden and Berkey's study. One very interesting feature of these authors' study was the survey conducted into the backgrounds of the fire-fighters. This showed that 55 per cent of the group 'indicated that as children their own fire-setting behaviour was no different from that of the average youngster'.[21] Moreover, 15 per cent of the group 'indicated that their children had played with fire against their wishes'.[22] The authors also concluded from their survey of fire-fighters that a not insignificant number of them suffered a great deal of stress and that this was revealed in such phenomena as high levels of family discord.

CONCLUSION

In this chapter I have sought to demonstrate that childhood fire-raising can best be understood by trying to formulate classfications, as I did with adult arsonists. This should facilitate management directed at the particular age level, social milieu and degree of disturbance in the young person. It is important that fire-raising behaviour in children should be taken seriously, however innocent it may appear. The evidence seems to indicate that 'large oaks from little acorns grow'. The recognition that we have a long way to go in educating young children and parents about the dangers of fire and in instituting preventive measures is of the greatest importance. This forms the subject of the concluding chapter.

7

WIDER ASPECTS OF MANAGEMENT AND PREVENTION

'Prevention is better than Cure.'
Proverb
'Dangers by being despised grow great.'
Edmund Burke, 'Speech on the Petition of the Unitarians'

INTRODUCTION

In previous chapters I have looked briefly at the manifestation of fire in various forms, particularly when used unlawfully, its detection, and more closely at the motives, attitudes and management at the individual level of those who engage in fire-raising activities. As I draft this chapter fire's potential for causing massive damage (and not a little controversy over who should foot the bill) is brought home to me sharply by the recent events at Windsor Castle. We know that the management of persistent fire-raisers presents considerable problems, particularly the question of how to predict further engagement in fire-raising by those who have already embarked upon it. Having said this, it is as well to recall, as indicated in Chapter 3, that arson constitutes a small percentage of all crimes of wilful damage in the UK; that said, it is *also* important to remember that a not inconsiderable number of cases of arson may go undetected. It is encouraging to note that only a small percentage of arsonists go on to repeat their crime, though, as with other criminal activity, we are not sure whether this is due to our interventive activities, or chance factors. However, it is also important to remember that a large proportion do go on to commit other offences. As indicated in Chapter 5, Sapsford *et al.* found that the reconviction rate of arsonists for *any criminal offence* was much higher than for other offenders – 80 per cent for offenders serving long sentences and 44 per cent for those with medium-term sentences.[1] In the survey of Social Enquiry Reports carried out by the Home Office Working Group on the Prevention of Arson, 13 per cent of the arsonists had been previously convicted of arson. As the authors of this report state: 'This is not a significant rate of re-offending if compared with other offences such as burglary, vehicle crime and (non-arson) criminal damage.'[2] However, before we take too much comfort from these figures, let us recall that arson can have the most devastating effects upon large numbers of victims and upon property. So far I have concentrated upon the perpetrators and said little, except *en passant*, about victims. The Working Group referred to above helps us to redress the balance; their views are worth quoting in full.

Supporting Victims of Arson

We believe that there is an unsatisfied demand for practical and emotional support for the victims of arson.

(43) We recommend that research be undertaken to ascertain the real needs of victims and the best ways to help them.

(44) We recommend that written guidance be provided to volunteers who help arson victims.

(45) We recommend that all arson victims should be given the option of referral to local victim support schemes and that both the police and the fire services should review their policies to ensure that this happens.

(46) We recommend that all arson attacks in which the victims or the community believe there is a racial motive need to be taken extremely seriously by the authorities. They need to make it clear to victims and to the community that they care about the attack and are doing something about it.

(47) We recommend that consideration should be given to the establishment of victim support schemes for businesses.

(48) We recommend that trade associations should take a much greater part in providing advice to their members to help them deal with the effects of arson or other serious incidents.[3]

In the light of the recent increase in arson attacks on minority groups referred to in Chapter 5, these recommendations assume an even greater importance than when they were promulgated some five years ago.

THE ACKNOWLEDGEMENT OF FIRE AS A HAZARD

Although concern with the psychopathology of the individual fire-raiser – adult or child – is important, it is also very necessary to place this in its social and historical context. As has been cogently pointed out,

> The use of fire, in its primitive forms, has become more forbidden and regulated as our society has become more urbanized. Citizens are no longer permitted to burn garbage and leaves on their property. Opportunities to build recreational camp-fires are now curtailed at most public parks and beaches.[4]

Although this quotation describes the situation in the United States, it is equally applicable to other communities. Children in particular are lacking opportunities to be exposed to the hazards of fire and to learn about avoiding its harmful effects. Central heating has replaced the open fire in many homes; little cooking now takes place upon the open hearth – modern cookers and the microwave have replaced it; rubbish-burning on a bonfire is prohibited more often than not. Many homes do not even have a fire-place, or, if they do, it is likely to be for 'cosmetic' effect only. One may speculate, therefore, that children are provided with less and less opportunity to experience the hazards (and delights) of fire under controlled conditions. Such lessening in exposure may make it even more mystifying and exciting; an allure created by its absence. We may also speculate on the extent to which the ready availability of fire services may have made us less conscious of the harmful effects of fire and bred a certain degree of contempt for its hazards. Wooden and Berkey highlight these speculations when they state:

> To the child of the past, who was taught to fear fire and was instructed in its proper use, we can compare the child of today, who may view a fire truck and sirens as fun and exciting. Or worse, he or she may view them as just another

form of entertainment (like watching action programs on television), having little, if any, comprehension of fire's danger to life and society.[5]

With the increase in fire-raising by children and young people, and the desire to make parents more accountable in law for their children's behaviour, questions have been asked as to the extent to which parents should be held responsible for the fire-raising activities of their offspring. A recent newspaper account describes an attempt by a local authority to 'lodge a claim for damages in the High Court against the families of two teenagers found guilty of setting fire to a school'. The chairman of the local education committee is stated to have said, in my view somewhat controversially, 'I don't see why parents should get away scot-free. If they leave their children out at night to set fire to a school there is no reason why they should not be in the dock with them' (*The Independent*, October 13, 1992, p. 2).

So far, our concentration has been on what might perhaps be called secondary preventive activity and focused very much upon the individual. It is now time to consider activities that might best be described as primary prevention – a macro- as distinct from a micro-approach, though the permeable boundaries between the two are acknowledged and were referred to in Chapter 1.

PRIMARY PREVENTIVE ACTIVITIES

I have already referred to the importance of educating children in the harmful effects of fire. It is obvious that more needs to be done in this area *before children take to fire-raising*. It is here that the media may have an important impact. In Chapter 4 I referred to the way in which many people – both young and old – gain their impressions of fires, fire detection and fire-fighting through television programmes, videos and films. It is necessary to reiterate here that portrayal of these subjects serves no good purpose if it only glamorises the phenomena. The Working Group on Arson make three very sensible recommendations on this matter. They state: 'That the portrayal of arson in the media may influence people and is likely to have a marked effect on the young.' They recommend:

That those in a position of responsibility in the media should recognise fully the opportunities and threats provided by this aspect of their work. We recommend that any reporting of arson should show the end of the story – highlighting police and court action, as well as the work of the fire services and the damage and heartache caused to the victims of arson. We recommend that those responsible for handling fictional material in the media should have a greater awareness of the impact on the public of the portrayal of arson.[6]

Woodward considers that despite the many problems presented by arson and arsonists 'the good news . . . is that it is at long last being recognized for the threat it is. The turning point was the symposium, organized in Brussels in November, 1985, by the CFPA [Conference of Fire Protection Associations of Europe]. This symposium, comprising high-level representatives from 14 countries, served for the first time to bring arson to the fore as an issue of importance to governments, police, fire services, insurers and other national bodies'.[7] A European working party has been established with the task of setting in train a 'comprehensive programme of counter-measures against arson'.[8] These counter-measures will include the following:

1 security measures – as a clear responsibility of management;
2 assessment of arson risk;
3 arson investigation;
4 guidance about fire protection equipment and security measures;
5 publicity and education;
6 community and local initiatives;
7 motivations of arsonists.

In addition, Woodward reports that national groups have been established with representation from, amongst others, the Home Office, the Home Office Forensic Science Service, the Fire Officers' Association, the Institution of Fire Engineers, the Association of Chief Police Officers, the Association of County Councils, the Association of British Insurers, the Chartered Institute of Loss Adjusters, the Fire Research Association and the Fire Protection Association.

As part of this continuing awareness and activity, it is encouraging to note the setting up early in 1991 of the Arson

Prevention Bureau (a joint venture by the Home Office and the Association of British Insurers). Its aims are 'to reduce arson by raising standards of fire investigation, collecting and disseminating information and best practice policies as well as promoting an arson prevention programme' (*The Independent*, February 18, 1991).

Much has been written and said about the vulnerability of victims; less is noted about the vulnerability of fire-fighters (though in Chapter 6 I made passing reference to the strains they may suffer). It was, therefore, of interest to note that the Health and Safety Executive recently issued a report which criticised the level of 'refresher' training given to firemen in the London Fire and Civil Defence Authority. This followed the deaths of two firemen in a south-east London fire in July 1991. The Health and Safety Executive wished for the lessons learned from their inquiry to be applied to all British fire brigades (*The Independent*, October 6, 1992).

WIDER ENVIRONMENTAL ISSUES

The prevention of fire-raising, particularly that which is vandalistic in motive, requires a broad perspective that embraces all forms of anti-social conduct, particularly in areas of great economic and social deprivation. In a recent well-argued paper Hope and Foster have illustrated very powerfully 'the socially harmful effects of concentrating [such] a large number of vulnerable people together in an already stressed environment'.[9] As long ago as 1980, a Home Office Working Party on Fires Caused by Vandalism suggested that 'the targets of fires caused by vandalism are very diverse but the risk of malicious ignition is higher in premises that are isolated, unattended and with little or no security and in those where children and young persons congregate'.[10] Their recommendations were, in summarised form, as follows:

1 better building design and modification to existing buildings;
2 education in vulnerability by use of alarms, sprinklers and detector systems;
3 better surveillance by all parties including the establishment of *ad hoc* patrols in high risk areas and specially appointed staff;
4 more care by owner-occupiers and better liaison between fire,

police and the insurance industry.[11]

A CONTEMPORARY PERSPECTIVE

The Arson Dossier, published in the UK by the Fire Protection Association, is the work of thirteen associations which comprise the Conference of Fire Protection Associations (CFPA). It contains a number of prescriptions for preventive activity; these are of recent date and may be summarised as follows:

1 *Security as part of management responsibility.* In a section entitled 'Approaches to a Solution', the authors state:

> The risk of arson in companies is of a different nature from other types of risk. The prevention strategy to be implemented must be both *original and imaginative* [italics added], and must be aimed at improving human relations and exchange of information in the company, since these two aspects are essential to the success of the strategy. This approach is particularly important in dealing with potential arson committed by persons working for, or having once worked for the company, whether their motivation is personal or dictated by factors outside the company, i.e. when an employee is used as an instrument.
>
> Prevention in this field must be centred on human relations and must concern every level of the company . . . . It would seem desirable to establish contact with the family, the family doctor and friends of a person identified as guilty of attempted arson, with the aim of understanding his motivation, giving him the best possible treatment and helping him back to normalcy.[12]

The statement then goes on to identify the roles that can be played in combatting arson by various grades of staff, such as managers, supervisory staff, security chiefs, employees and trade unions.

2 *Security measures.* These build upon the previous recommendations by a number of bodies, such as the Home Office Working Party on Fires Caused by Vandalism referred to above. They include the following:
    (a) adequate enclosure of buildings;

   (b) building security;
   (c) adequate lighting;
   (d) surveillance systems;
   (e) storage of combustibles, good standards of cleanliness and tidiness;
   (f) guarding of premises at vulnerable times.

3 *Building design.* Various suggestions are made for improvement such as good visibility, dangers inherent in flat roofs, unsupervised possible escape routes and clear, uncluttered lay-out of buildings.

4 *Fire protection equipment.* Warning and detection systems are recommended.

5 *Community action and local initiatives against arson.* These can be implemented at national, regional and local levels. In the *Arson Dossier*, the recommendations are based upon practice in Sweden, but they are quite applicable in other countries. They suggest the following forms of activity, amongst others:
   (a) Bringing together *all* interested parties and organisations.
   (b) Study of arson patterns and trends.
   (c) Development of information systems and procedures. They advocate the establishment of 'arson clubs' for the dissemination of views and information.

In the UK four kinds of regional groups are engaged in fire safety and fire-fighting: (i) fire liaison panels, (ii) local fire protection associations, (iii) an Industrial Fire Protection Association and (iv) crime prevention panels with a special focus on arson.

Anyone interested in the broader aspects of fire prevention, and arson in particular, would do well to study the *Arson Dossier*. In addition to the *Dossier*, the Fire Protection Association has produced a series of most informative booklets and leaflets on fire safety, investigation and case illustrations of arson attacks.

CONCLUSION

Much of the foregoing material has concerned itself with the need for adequate publicity and education at both the micro- and macro-levels. The preventive measures that can be taken to combat fire-raising in its many forms have also been described. The compilers of the *Arson Dossier* have a very sober message to convey concerning the role of education and publicity:

> In compiling information and publicity . . . it is important
> not to over-exaggerate the threat which may have the effect
> of causing people to feel that nothing can usefully be
> achieved. The provision of sober, factual information is
> clearly the right approach for the responsible managements
> in industrial, commercial and public buildings (e.g.
> schools). However, even for these categories of people,
> bearing in mind that many of them still remain ignorant of
> the very real threat which arson poses, an occasional
> reminder in more dramatic terms is also required.[13]

To this one would merely wish to add that although a study of the
psychopathology of arsonists is vital, their behaviour must be
viewed in a broad social and political context. If my modest
survey of the problem has aided understanding along the lines
suggested in the quotation above and has avoided the dangers of
over-dramatic presentation, it will have achieved its aim.

NOTES AND REFERENCES

1 PREAMBLE

1 M. Douglas, *Purity and Danger: An Analysis of the Concepts of Pollution and Taboo*, London, Ark Books, 1984, p. 138.
2 See D. Scott, *Fire and Fire-Raisers*, London, Duckworth, 1974; D. Canter (ed.), *Fires and Human Behaviour*, Chichester, John Wiley, 1980. For US accounts see J.M. Macdonald, *Bombers and Firesetters*, Springfield, Ill., Charles C. Thomas, 1977, and W.S. Wooden and M.L. Berkey, *Children and Arson: America's Middle Class Nightmare*, New York and London, Plenum Press, 1984.

2 CONTEXT

1 J. Bronowski, *The Ascent of Man*, London, BBC, 1976, p. 124.
2 See H. Prins, *Bizarre Behaviours: Boundaries of Psychiatry*, London, Tavistock/Routledge, 1990, Chapter 5. For a more detailed recent account of the phenomenon in literature see C. Frayling, *Vampyres: Lord Byron to Count Dracula*, London, Faber & Faber, 1991.
3 See D.O. Topp, 'Fire as a Symbol and as a Weapon of Death', *Medicine, Science and the Law*, Vol. 13, 1973, p. 79 (pp. 79–86).
4 Ibid.
5 See, for example, R.H. Robbins, *The Encyclopaedia of Witchcraft and Demonology*, London, Newnes Books, 1984.
6 Sir J.G. Frazer, *The Golden Bough: A Study in Magic and Religion* (abridged edn), London, Macmillan, 1987. First published in 1922 in twelve volumes.
7 Ibid., p. 64.
8 Ibid., p. 615.
9 C. Hole, *A Dictionary of British Folk Customs*, London, Paladin, 1978.
10 Ibid., p. 53.
11 Ibid., p. 50.
12 J.M. Macdonald, *Bombers and Firesetters*, Springfield, Ill., Charles C. Thomas, 1977, p. 9.
13 Ibid.

14 D. Scott, *Fire and Fire-Raisers*, London, Duckworth, 1974, p. 6.
15 Ibid.

3 THE SIZE OF THE PROBLEM AND LEGAL ASPECTS

1 Home Office, *Report of Working Party on Fires Caused by Vandalism*, London, 1980.
2 G.B. Palermo, M.B. Smith, J.J. Dinotto and T.P. Christopher, 'Victimization Revisited: A National Statistical Analysis', *International Journal of Offender Therapy and Comparative Criminology*, Vol. 36, 1991, pp. 187–201.
3 A. Lewis, 'Future Developments in the Battle Against Arson', *Fire Prevention*, Vol. 216, 1989, pp. 36–40.
4 A. Storr, *Human Destructiveness: The Roots of Genocide and Human Cruelty* (second edn), London, Routledge, 1991, pp. 141–2.
5 C.D. Woodward, 'Arson: The Major Fire Problem of the 1980s', *Journal of the Society of Fellows. The Chartered Insurance Institute*, Vol. 2 (Pt 1), 1987, pp. 55–68.
6 Ibid., p. 55.
7 Ibid.
8 Small fires (as distinct from those defined as 'large') are those affecting single derelict buildings, a single tree, an outdoor fire confined to grassland, heath, railway embankments, fences, derelict cars, road surfaces, telegraph poles, etc. Home Office, *Standing Conference on Crime Prevention: Report of the Working Group on the Prevention of Arson*, London, December 6, 1988, p. 83. The Glossary in this report has some helpful definitions. For example, deliberate/possibly deliberate fires are defined as follows. A *deliberate* fire is one where the fire brigade records that malicious or deliberate ignition is established beyond reasonable doubt. A *possibly deliberate* fire is one where malicious or deliberate ignition is merely suspected. The fire services record such fires as of 'doubtful defect, act or omission'. An occupied building is one which is in use (i.e. not derelict). *It need not have people in it at the time of the fire* (p. 83).
9 Apart from the year 1986, a clearly discernible rise can be noted. However, it should also be observed that although arson and criminal damage endangering life are very serious crimes, they only constitute about 2 per cent of all offences against property as revealed in the criminal statistics. Serious cases of arson and criminal damage endangering life are normally dealt with by custodial penalties. In 1984, for example, of 2,491 persons found guilty of arson, 799 received immediate custodial penalties (Woodward, op. cit., p. 56).
10 The special hospitals in England and Wales are established under statute for persons subject to detention under the mental health legislation who require treatment in conditions of high security because of their dangerous, violent or criminal propensities. (Section 4, National Health Service Act, 1977.) Scotland's equivalent is the State Hospital at Carstairs and Southern Ireland's equivalent is

Dublin's Central Dundrum Hospital. There is no similar provision for Northern Ireland; the latter places a small number of its dangerous patients in England and Wales.

11 Statistics supplied by courtesy of the Special Hospitals Service Authority. I am grateful to Mr Martin Butwell, Data Base Manager, for his assistance. Any errors of interpretation are mine.

12 Information kindly supplied in correspondence by Mr J.C. Munro, Secretary to the Crime Insurance Panel of the Association of British Insurers, October 4, 1990.

13 Home Office Research and Statistics Department, *Fire Statistics 1988 United Kingdom*, London, 1990, p. 12. For anyone wishing to secure a detailed picture of the nature and extent of fires from all causes throughout the UK these annual statistics are a most useful source of information.

14 All statistics below taken from ibid.

15 A non-fatal casualty is defined as an instance of a person requiring medical treatment beyond first aid given at the scene of the fire or needing to be taken to hospital, or advised to see a doctor for check-up or observation (ibid., p. 110).

16 Unascribed report in *Fire Engineering*, January 1990, p. 24.

17 Ibid.

18 J.W. Bradford, 'Arson: A Review', in M.H. Ben-Aron, S.J. Hucker and C.D. Webster (eds), *Clinical Criminology: The Assessment and Treatment of Criminal Behaviour*, Toronto, Clarke Institute of Psychiatry, 1985.

19 Information below taken from Woodward, op. cit. pp. 57–9.

20 Ibid., pp. 59–61.

21 J.L. Geller, 'Pathological Fire-setting in Adults', *International Journal of Law and Psychiatry*, Vol. 15, 1992, pp. 283–302. Those readers interested in exploring the criteria that determined whether one was hanged or suffered some other form of execution could usefully consult G. Abbott, *Lords of the Scaffold: A History of the Executioner*, London, Robert Hale, and New York, St Martin's Press, 1991.

22 Mr R.D. Mackay, Reader in Criminal Law, De Montfort University, Leicester. Letter to the author, October 21, 1992.

4 THE INVESTIGATION OF FIRE-RAISING

1 R.A. Cooke and R.H. Ide, *Principles of Fire Investigation*, Leicester, Institution of Fire Engineers, 1985 (notably Chapters 4, 6, 10, 15, 16, 21 and 24). Aspects of human behaviour in fires and fire hazards are dealt with usefully in D. Canter (ed.), *Fires and Human Behaviour*, Chichester, John Wiley, 1980 (notably in Chapters 5, 6, 8, 9 and 10).

2 N.F. Richards, 'Fire Investigation – Destruction of Corpses', *Medicine, Science and the Law*, Vol. 17, 1977, pp. 79–82.

3 CPFA Europe, *Arson Dossier* (UK edn), London, Fire Protection Association, n.d.

4 In the UK, fire service staff receive nationally based training in the basics of fire investigation at the Fire Service College, Moreton-in-Marsh, Gloucestershire. A degree of local training also takes place.

5 Annex A to circular.
6 C. Clisby, in D. Canter (ed.), op. cit., p. 323.
7 C.D. Woodward, 'Arson: The Major Fire Problem of the 1980s', *Journal of the Society of Fellows. The Chartered Insurance Institute*, Vol. 2 (Pt 1), 1987, p. 61 (pp. 55–68).
8 J.M. Macdonald, *Bombers and Firesetters*, Springfield, Ill., Charles C. Thomas, 1977.
9 Cooke and Ide, op. cit., pp. 398–9.
10 Ibid., p. 160.
11 Ibid., pp. 160–1.
12 CPFA Europe, op. cit., p. 21.

5 ADULT FIRE-RAISERS: MOTIVES AND MANAGEMENT

1 See, for example, H. Prins, 'Mental Abnormality and Criminality – An Uncertain Relationship', *Medicine, Science and the Law*, Vol. 30, 1990, pp. 247–58, and more recently an extended treatment by S. Wessely and P.J. Taylor, 'Madness and Crime: Criminology versus Psychiatry', *Criminal Behaviour and Mental Health*, Vol. 1, 1991, pp. 193–228.
2 H. Prins, G. Tennent, and K. Trick, 'Motives for Arson (Fire-Raising)', *Medicine, Science and the Law*, Vol. 25, 1985, pp. 275–8.
3 K. Soothill, 'Arson', in R. Bluglass and P. Bowden (eds), *Principles and Practice of Forensic Psychiatry*, London and Edinburgh, Churchill Livingstone, 1990, p. 782.
4 Ibid.
5 W.S. Wooden and M.L. Berkey, *Children and Arson: America's Middle Class Nightmare*, New York and London, Plenum Press, 1984.
6 Home Office, *Standing Conference on Crime Prevention: Report of the Working Group on the Prevention of Arson*, London, December 6, 1988, p. 41 (italics added).
7 J.M. Macdonald, *Bombers and Firesetters*, Springfield, Ill., Charles C. Thomas, 1977, p. 242.
8 Soothill, op. cit., p. 780.
9 R. Rendel, *Kissing the Gunner's Daughter*, London, Arrow Books, 1992, p. 315.
10 J.A. Inciardi, 'The Adult Firesetter: A Typology', *Criminology*, Vol. 8, August 1970, pp. 145–55.
11 J. Ravateheino, 'Finnish Study of 180 Arsonists Arrested in Helsinki', *Fire Protection*, Vol. 223, 1989, pp. 30–4.
12 M. Faulk, *Basic Forensic Psychiatry*, Oxford, Blackwell Scientific Publications, 1988, pp. 91–7.
13 The original classification in Prins et al., op. cit., has been modified slightly for present purposes.
14 Home Office, *Report of the Working Group on the Prevention of Arson*, op. cit., p. 72.
15 R.A. Cooke and R.H. Ide, *Principles of Fire Investigation*, Leicester, The Institution of Fire Engineers, 1985, esp. Chapter 16, pp. 248–60.

16 This chapter and the next contain a number of case illustrations. Where these are derived from materials in the public domain (such as newspaper accounts), no attempt has been made at disguise – other than by not naming the offender. In cases drawn from my own professional experience, significant identifying data have been altered so as to preserve anonymity. In some instances 'composite' cases are presented. However, such necessary and important disguises do not invalidate the relevance or significance of the material.

17 There are a number of useful studies of the general characteristics of arsonists. The classic study is that by N.D.C. Lewis and H. Yarnell, *Pathological Firesetting (Pyromania)*, Nervous and Mental Disease Monographs, No. 82, New York, Coolidge Foundation, 1951. This examined the characteristics of more than 1,000 young arsonists; unfortunately no control group was used. In an earlier study, Yarnell found a high proportion of child arsonists had serious learning problems. See H. Yarnell, 'Firesetting in Children', *American Journal of Orthopsychiatry*, Vol. 10, 1940, pp. 262–86. For examples of surveys of imprisoned and hospitalised arsonists see W. Hurley and T.M. Monahan, 'Arson: The Criminal and the Crime', *British Journal of Criminology*, Vol. 9, 1969, pp. 4–21, G.H. O'Sullivan and M.J. Kelleher, 'A Study of Firesetters in the South-West of Ireland', *British Journal of Psychiatry*, Vol. 151, 1987, pp. 818–23. A survey of psychological aspects may be found in R.G. Vreeland and B.M. Levin, 'Psychological Aspects of Fire-Setting', in D. Canter (ed.), *Fires and Human Behaviour*, Chichester, John Wiley, 1980. For studies of special hospital populations see D.W. McKerracher and A.J.I. Dacre, 'A Study of Arsonists in a Special Security Hospital', *British Journal of Psychiatry*, Vol. 112, 1966, pp. 1151–4, and T.G. Tennent, A. McQuaid, T. Loughnane and A.J. Hands, 'Female Arsonists', *British Journal of Psychiatry*, Vol. 119, 1971, pp. 497–502. The recidivism of arsonists is dealt with in K.L. Soothill and P.J. Pope, 'Arson: A Twenty-Year Cohort Study', *Medicine, Science and the Law*, Vol. 13, 1973, pp. 127–38, and in R.J. Sapsford, C. Banks and D.D. Smith, 'Arsonists in Prison', *Medicine, Science and the Law*, Vol. 18, 1978, pp. 247–54. A more detailed recent account of the interpersonal functioning of arsonists may be found in H.F. Jackson, S. Hope and C. Glass, 'Why are Arsonists not Violent Offenders?', *International Journal of Offender Therapy and Comparative Criminology*, Vol. 31, 1987, pp. 143–51. The need to review family dynamics is stated clearly by Regehr and Glancy; see C. Regehr and G. Glancy, 'Families of Firesetters', *The Journal of Forensic Psychiatry*, Vol. 2, 1991, pp. 27–36.

18 Cooke and Ide, op. cit., p. 248.

19 Dr K. Rix, Senior Lecturer, Department of Psychiatry, Leeds University. Paper given to Royal College of Psychiatrists' Spring Meeting, Leeds, April 1989.

20 Cooke and Ide, op. cit. See also Macdonald, op. cit., p. 197.

21 Cooke and Ide, op. cit., p. 251.

22 C.D. Woodward, 'Arson: The Major Fire Problem of the 1980s',

Journal of the Society of Fellows. The Chartered Insurance Institute, Vol. 2 (Pt 1), 1987, pp. 55–68.

23 Ibid., p. 64.

24 Quoted in E. Barker, *New Religious Movements: A Practical Introduction*, London, HMSO, 1989, pp. 54–5.

25 D.O. Topp, 'Fire as a Symbol and as a Weapon of Death', *Medicine, Science and the Law*, Vol. 13, 1973, pp. 79–86.

26 J. Newton, 'Suicide by Fire', *Medicine, Science and the Law*, Vol. 16, 1976, pp. 177–9.

27 Quoted in G. Abbott, *Lords of the Scaffold: A History of the Executioner*, London, Robert Hale, and New York, St Martin's Press, 1991, p. 167.

28 For a summary of the characteristics of the main mental disorders see H. Prins, *Offenders, Deviants or Patients: An Introduction to the Study of Socio-Forensic Problems*, London, Tavistock, 1980.

29 M. Virkunnen, 'On Arson Committed by Schizophrenics', *Acta Psychiatrica Scandinavica*, Vol. 50, 1974, pp. 152–4.

30 D. Scott, *Fire and Fire-Raisers*, London, Duckworth, 1974, Chapter 11.

31 Soothill, op. cit., p. 785. The standard reference work on Martin seems to be T. Balston, *The Life of Jonathan Martin: Incendiarist of York Minster*, London, Macmillan, 1945.

32 Hurley and Monahan, op. cit.

33 P.K. Carpenter and A.L. King, 'Epilepsy and Arson', *British Journal of Psychiatry*, Vol. 154, 1989, pp. 554–6.

34 A. Byrne and J.B. Walsh, Letter, 'The Epileptic Arsonist', *British Journal of Psychiatry*, Vol. 155, 1989, p. 268.

35 McKerracher and Dacre, op. cit.

36 The Mental Health Act, 1983, in addition to giving courts power to make orders for treatment in hospitals of various kinds, also enables the Home Secretary to transfer persons either serving a sentence or on remand to hospital provided that the criteria of the Act are satisfied. In brief, this means that they are stated by two doctors approved under the Act to be suffering from one or other of the forms of mental disorder named in the Act and that they require treatment in hospital for their own protection or that of others. If a crown court considers that the public needs to be protected from serious harm it may add to a hospital order an order restricting discharge either for a finite period or without time limit. For those unfamiliar with the legislation a summarised account may be found in my book *Dangerous Behaviour, the Law and Mental Disorder*, London, Tavistock, 1986, Chapter 3.

37 K. Thomas, *Religion and the Decline of Magic: Studies in Popular Beliefs in Sixteenth- and Seventeenth-Century England*, Harmondsworth Penguin Books, 1984, p. 634.

38 Ibid., p. 636.

39 Ibid., p. 635.

40 Woodward, op. cit., p. 62.

41 See Soothill and Pope, op. cit.

42 J.L. Geller, J. Erlen and R.L. Pinkus, 'A Historical Appraisal of America's Experience with "Pyromania" – a Diagnosis in Search of a

Disorder', *International Journal of Law and Psychiatry*, Vol. 9, 1986, pp. 201–29.

43 H. Maudsley, *Responsibility in Mental Disease*, New York, D. Appleton and Co., p. 81 (Quoted in Geller *et al.*, op. cit., p. 208).

44 W. Stekel, *Peculiarities of Behaviour*, New York, Boni and Liveright, 1924.

45 Geller *et al.*, op. cit., p. 223.

46 American Psychiatric Association, *Diagnostic and Statistical Manual of Mental Disorders* (third edn – revised), New York, 1987, p. 325.

47 Ibid.

48 Quoted in Vreeland and Levin, op. cit., fn. 13.

49 J.L. Geller, 'Pathological Fire-setting in Adults', *International Journal of Law and Psychiatry*, Vol. 15, 1992, p. 292 (pp. 283–302).

50 D.W. Winnicott, *Collected Papers: Through Paediatrics to Psycho-Analysis*, London, Tavistock, 1958, Chapter XXV, p. 309.

51 M.E. Rice and G.T. Harris, 'Mentally Disordered Firesetters', *Penetanguishene Mental Health Centre Research Report*, Vol. 1, No. 2, Ontario, March 1984.

52 L.J. Foust, 'The Legal Significance of Clinical Formulations of Firesetting', *International Journal of Law and Psychiatry*, Vol. 2, 1979, pp. 371–87.

53 I. Fras, 'Fire Setting (Pyromania) and Its Relationship to Sexuality', in L.B. Schlesinger and E. Revitch (eds), *Sexual Dynamics of Anti-Social Behaviour*, Springfield, Ill., Charles C. Thomas, 1983, p. 199.

54 Ibid.

55 Hurley and Monahan, op. cit.

56 E. Simmel, 'Incendiarism', in K.R. Eissler (ed.), *Searchlights on Delinquency: New Psychoanalytic Studies*, London, Imago Publishing Co., 1949.

57 Ibid., p. 95.

58 Ibid., p. 96.

59 Cooke and Ide, op. cit., p. 252.

60 A. Storr, *Human Destructiveness: The Roots of Genocide and Human Cruelty* (second edn), London, Routledge, 1991, p. 143.

61 M. Faulk, 'The Assessment of Dangerousness in Arsonists', in. J.R. Hamilton and H. Freeman (eds), *Dangerousness: Psychiatric Assessment and Management*, London, Gaskell Books, for Royal College of Psychiatrists, 1982, p. 72.

62 Department of Health and Home Office, *Review of Health and Social Services for Mentally Disordered Offenders* (Reed Committee, various reports), London, 1992.

63 M. Cox, *Structuring the Therapeutic Process: Compromise with Chaos – the Therapists's Response to the Individual and the Group*, Oxford, Pergamon, 1978, p. 140.

64 M. Cox, 'Dynamic Psychotherapy With Sex-Offenders', in. I. Rosen (ed.), *Sexual Deviation* (second edn), Oxford, Oxford University Press, 1979, p. 320.

65 Ibid., p. 332.

66 Ibid., p. 334.

67 Ibid., p. 344.
68 Jackson *et al.*, op. cit.
69 Ibid., p. 151.
70 G.T. Harris and M.E. Rice, 'Mentally Disordered Firesetters: Psychodynamic versus Empirical Approaches', *International Journal of Law and Psychiatry*, Vol. 7, 1984, pp. 19–34.
71 I.C.H. Clare, G.H. Murphy, D. Cox and E.H. Chaplin, 'Assessment and Treatment of Fire-Setting: A Single-case Investigation Using a Cognitive-Behavioural Model', *Criminal Behaviour and Mental Health*, Vol. 2, 1992, pp. 253–68.
72 Ibid., p. 266.
73 Faulk, op. cit, p. 74.
74 H. Prins, *Dangerous Behaviour, the Law and Mental Disorder*, London, Tavistock, 1986; 'Up in Smoke! The Psychology of Arson', *Medico-Legal Journal*, Vol. 55, 1987, pp. 69–84; 'Dangerous People or Dangerous Situations? – Some Further Thoughts', *Medicine, Science and the Law*, Vol. 31, 1991, pp. 25–37.
75 P.D. Scott, 'Assessing Dangerousness in Criminals', *British Journal of Psychiatry*, Vol. 131, 1977, pp. 127–42.
76 Ibid., p. 129.

6 CHILD FIRE-RAISERS: MOTIVES AND MANAGEMENT

1 H. Yarnell, 'Firesetting in Children', *American Journal of Orthopsychiatry*, Vol. 10, 1940, pp. 262–86, N.D.C. Lewis and H. Yarnell, *Pathological Firesetting (Pyromania)*, Nervous and Mental Disease Monographs, No. 82, New York, Coolidge Foundation, 1951. No attempt is made here to review the literature comprehensively. Some helpful references are: B. Nurcombe, 'Children Who Set Fires', *Medical Journal of Australia*, April 18, 1964, pp. 579–84; K.R. Fineman, 'Firesetting in Childhood and Adolescence', *Psychiatric Clinics of North America*, Vol. 3, 1984, pp. 483–500; E.R. Bumpass, F.D. Fogelman and R.J. Brix, 'Intervention with Children Who Set Fires', *American Journal of Psychotherapy*, Vol. 37, 1983, pp. 328–45. W.S. Wooden and M.L. Berkey's *Children and Arson: America's Middle Class Nightmare*, New York and London, Plenum Press, 1984, also contains extensive references to the literature.
2 D. Kafry, 'Playing with Matches: Children and Fire', in D. Canter (ed.), *Fires and Human Behaviour*, Chichester, John Wiley, 1980.
3 Lewis and Yarnell, op. cit., p. 285.
4 M.A. Stewart and K.W. Culver, 'Children Who Set Fires: The Clinical Picture and a Follow-Up', *British Journal of Psychiatry*, Vol. 140, 1982, pp. 357–63. See also J.G. Strachan, 'Conspicuous Firesetting in Children', *British Journal of Psychiatry*, Vol. 138, 1981, pp. 26–9.
5 R. Jacobson, 'Child Firesetters: A Clinical Investigation', *Journal of Child Psychology and Psychiatry*, Vol. 26, 1985, pp. 759–68, and 'The Sub-Classification of Child Firesetters', *Journal of Child Psychology and Psychiatry*, Vol. 26, 1985, pp. 769–75.

6 I.P. Everall and A. LeCouteur, 'Fire-setting in a Boy with Asperger's Syndrome', *British Journal of Psychiatry*, Vol. 157, 1990, pp. 284–7.
7 L.B. Macht and J.E. Mack, 'The Firesetter Syndrome', *Psychiatry*, Vol. 31, 1968, pp. 277–88.
8 T.A. Vandersall and J.M. Wiener, 'Children Who Set Fires', *Archives of General Psychiatry*, Vol. 22, 1970, pp. 63–71.
9 Stewart and Culver, op. cit., p. 363.
10 G.A. Heath, W.F. Gayton and V.A. Hardesty, 'Childhood Firesetting', *Canadian Psychiatric Association Journal*, Vol. 21, 1976, p. 236 (pp. 229–37). It should be noted that there have been some significant studies of delinquent behaviours in childhood as precursors of adult criminality. See, for example, L.N. Robins, *Deviant Children Grown Up: A Sociological and Psychiatric Study of Sociopathic Personality*, Baltimore, Williams and Wilkins, 1966; D.J. West, *Delinquency, Its Roots, Careers and Prospects*, London, Heinemann, 1982. (This latter volume summarises the long-term research known as 'The Cambridge Study of Delinquent Development', previously published in three volumes, and numerous papers in learned journals.) The current state of the art in the UK is described succinctly by David P. Farrington in 'Criminal Career Research in the United Kingdom', *British Journal of Criminology*, Vol. 32, 1992, pp. 521–36.
11 Heath *et al.*, op. cit., p. 235.
12 Wooden and Berkey, op. cit. (n. 1).
13 Ibid., p. 4.
14 Kafry, op. cit. (n. 2).
15 In the article in question reference is also made to his autobiography, *Travelling Player*, London, Headline Press, 1991.
16 Wooden and Berkey, op. cit., p. 51.
17 A lengthy article written by Emily Green.
18 C.J. Holland, 'Elimination of Firesetting in a Seven-Year-Old Boy', *Behaviour Research and Therapy*, Vol. 7, 1969, pp. 135–7.
19 R.S. Welsh, 'The Use of Stimulus Satiation in the Elimination of Juvenile Firesetting Behaviour', in A.M. Graziano (ed.), *Behaviour Therapy with Children*, Chicago, Aldine Publishing, 1971.
20 S. Minuchin, *Families and Family Therapy*, London, Tavistock, 1977, Chapter 11.
21 Wooden and Berkey, op. cit., p. 150.
22 Ibid., p. 152.

7 WIDER ASPECTS OF MANAGEMENT AND PREVENTION

1 R.J. Sapsford, C. Banks, and D.D. Smith, 'Arsonists in Prison', *Medicine, Science and the Law*, Vol. 18, 1978, pp. 247–54.
2 Home Office, *Standing Conference on Crime Prevention: Report of the Working Group on the Prevention of Arson*, London, December 6, 1988, p. 42.
3 Ibid., p. 7.

4 W.S. Wooden and M.L. Berkey, *Children and Arson: American's Middle Class Nightmare*, New York and London, Plenum Books, 1984, p. 16.
5 Ibid., p. 18.
6 Home Office, *Report of the Working Group on Arson*, op. cit., pp. 5–6.
7 C.D. Woodward, 'Arson: The Major Fire Problem of the 1980s', *Journal of the Society of Fellows. The Chartered Insurance Institute*, Vol. 2 (Pt 1), 1987, p. 64 (pp. 55–68).
8 Ibid., p. 65.
9 T. Hope and J. Foster, 'Conflicting Forces: Changing the Dynamics of Crime and Community on a "Problem" Estate', *British Journal of Criminology*, Vol. 32, 1992, p. 501 (pp. 488–504).
10 Home Office, *Report of Working Party on Fires Caused by Vandalism*, London, 1980, p. 19.
11 Ibid., p. 20.
12 CFPA Europe, *Arson Dossier*, (UK edn), London, Fire Protection Association, n.d., pp. 23–4.
13 Ibid., p. 44.

FURTHER READING

Some of the works listed below have already been referred to in the text. They are referred to again here because they contain additional material which may be of interest to readers.

The Arson Prevention Bureau, *Arson in Schools, Arson Update*, London, January 1993.

D. Canter (ed.) *Fires and Human Behaviour*, Chichester, John Wiley, 1980.

Fire Protection Association, London, *Arson Bibliography*, January 1989. (Contains an international bibliography on the psychology of arson, fire investigation, juvenile fire-raising and a list of foreign language papers.)

Fire Research Station, *References to Literature on Arson and Incendiarism*, Library Bibliography, No. 180 (July 1979) and *Supplement* No. 1 (June 1992), Elstree, Middlesex.

Gerling Institute, *Arson*, Cologne, 1983.

Home Office (Fire Department), *Fires Caused by Vandalism: Summary of Proceedings of a Home Office Seminar*, April 1–2, 1980.

National Institute of Law Enforcement and Criminal Justice, *Arson: A Selected Bibliography*, United States Department of Justice, Washington, January 1979.

A.O. Rider, 'The Firesetter: A Psychological Profile' (Parts I and II), *International Police Review*, May and June/July 1984.

W.S. Wooden and M.L. Berkey, *Children and Arson: America's Middle Class Nightmare*, New York and London, Plenum Press, 1984.

SOME RELEVANT JOURNALS

British Journal of Criminology
British Journal of Psychiatry
Criminal Behaviour and Mental Health
Fire
Fire Engineering
Fire Journal
Fire Prevention
Fire Protection Review
The Journal of Forensic Psychiatry
Medicine, Science and the Law

NAME INDEX

Abbott, Elizabeth 57

Barker, E. 47
Berkey, M.L. 3, 36, 79–82, 84–5, 88–9
Bradford, J.W. 23
Bronowski, J. 4
Burke, Edmund 86
Butwell, Martin 97 n.11
Byrne, A. 53, 68

Campbell, Angus 63
Canter, D. 3
Carpenter, P.K. 53, 68
Clare, I.C.H. 71–2
Clisby, Charles 30
Cooke, R.A. 28, 29, 31, 32, 40, 43
Cox, M. 69–71
Culver, K.W. 77, 78–9

Da Vinci, Leonardo 9
Dacre, A.J.I. 54
Day, Sir Michael vii–viii
Douglas, Mary 1

Eco, Umberto 4
Everall, I.P. 77–8

Faulk, M. 37–9, 68, 73
Foster, Anne 57
Foster, J. 91
Foust, L.J. 63
Fras, I. 64
Frazer, Sir James George 6–9

Freud, Sigmund 6, 10, 61, 63

Geller, J.L. 25, 61, 62

Harris, G.T. 63, 71
Heath, G.A. 79
Hippocrates 9
Hole, Christina 8
Holland, C.J. 83
Hope, T. 91
Hurley, W. 52, 64

Ide, R.H. 28, 29, 31, 32, 40, 43
Inciardi, J.A. 37

Jackson, H.F. 71
Jacobson, R. 77
Jung, C.G. 6, 10, 61

Kafry, Ditsa 76–7, 80
King. A.L. 53, 68

LeCouteur, A. 77–8
Lee, Ronnie 45
Lewis, N.D.C. 62, 76, 79, 99 n.17

Macdonald, J.M. 3, 9, 30–1, 37
Macht, L.B. 78
Mack, J.E. 78
Mackay, R.D. 26
McKerracher, D.W. 54
McNaghten, Daniel 35–6
Marc 10
Martin, Jonathan 50–2

SUBJECT INDEX

111